*Secrets Beyond Your Plate for a
Healthier, More Energetic Life*

THE
G.U.T.
METHOD®

Sharon Holand Gelfand, CN

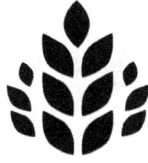

PRAISE FOR THE
G.U.T. METHOD

"Want to stop the diet merry-go-round? *The G.U.T. Method* is the book we have been waiting for, and the answers are here. Sharon Holand Gelfand talked to my tortured soul, tortured by years of dieting and not getting results. The G.U.T. Method breaks the cycle of diet obsession with a simple and effective plan for a new and healthy life. This book is revolutionary. Anyone who has ever been on a diet needs to read the groundbreaking *GU.T. Method*."

—*Dr. Betsy A.B. Greenleaf, DO, FACOOG (Distinguished), FACOG, MBA, premiere wellness expert and first U.S. board certified female urogynecologist*

"As a curvy, full-figured diva, I must admit that I have struggled with my weight in my thirties and forties. I can never commit to a diet, so I don't. I eat as I wish and lately, I have been feeling sluggish. Reading this book has led to an epiphany for me. The answers are in me and not in some guru's words. Sharon has demonstrated the frustration and irritation most of us feel when it comes to our bodies, health and life. In the first few pages alone, I found her talking to me from the pages, hearing and answering my questions.

What a great book for anyone ready to get off the diet merry-go-round. So necessary even in times like this! Two thumbs up!"

—*Precious L. Williams, CEO, Perfect Pitches by*
  Precious, LLC

"Sharon Holand Gelfand is one of the 'GUT-siest' people I know! Triggered by a personal health crisis, she dove headfirst into exploring the world of nutrition and food-related health issues, and in a short time, emerged as a top thought leader in this crucially important field. In this important and captivating book, not only does her extensive knowledge shine through, but so does her sense of passion and purpose in making it her mission to ensure that others lead healthier and, thus, happier lives. If the saying is true that, 'you are what you eat,' then it may also be true that 'you are what you read.' And, if so, I encourage you to have the G.U.T.S. to open this book…and your mind, as well as your heart (and your mouth), and digest this author's insightful and powerful advice. Doing so can, literally, save your life."

—*Todd Cherches, CEO, BigBlueGumball, author*
  of VisuaLeadership: Leveraging the Power of Visual
  Thinking in Leadership and in Life

"Reading about your microbiome and gut health sounds about as sexy as reading about politics. However, Sharon Holand Gelfand has found a way to share the truth about what's going on inside our insides in a way that is relatable, humorous and educational. Let's hope we can fix our guts and politics all at the same time!"

—*Tricia Brouk, international award-winning director*

"This book is a holistic, comprehensive pathway upon which Sharon guides you into a deep engagement with your optimum health and wellness. Science is unfolding studies of the gut as our second brain and this book will give you practical information and helpful ways in rebalancing and reaching your optimum health. Sharon writes with a practical and interesting narrative, which will enable real change for those who read this and follow the healthy way of being."

—*Diana Guy, leading expert in the study and applications of yoga and holistic health*

"Sharon Holand Gelfand is one-of-a-kind! She brings her talent, knowledge and passion to The G.U.T. Method and changes the conversation about health, nutrition, and dieting. This is the book to read! Your 'gut' is so much more than your belly. It is your health central station and Sharon has a unique way of enlightening all of us to think differently about the foods we eat and how to tune into how we feel. This book is not just a book about nutrition and how to eat well. It is a powerful book that will make you throw away your scale and get connected."

—*Robin Joy Meyers, TEDx speaker, molecular geneticist, author of* Alone, but Not Lonely: Reclaim Your

Identity and Be Unapologetically You! *and founder of the FEAR Method*

"Through fascinating historical accounts as well as her own personal experiences, Sharon takes the reader on a journey through the labyrinth that is the world of counting calories and shows the reader the truth: That the answer is not in some pill or food fad; it's within ourselves. If you're ready to cut the strings to the puppetry of doctors, drugs, and diets then pick up this book."

—*Michael Roderick, CEO, Small Pond Enterprises*

CONTENTS

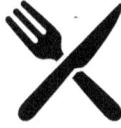

FOREWORD

Getting started is the greatest challenge of all. I know this to be true as I myself have "started" countless times! There have been periods in life when I've felt great and others when I've struggled. Times when I have felt empowered, and other times when I have felt totally lost. Life has ebbed and flowed, and I have expanded and contracted along with it. Perhaps you can relate.

What we know about health and nutrition is everchanging—our resources, our motivation, and how it all comes together, make our individual journeys unique. Perhaps this is why there are so many approaches to diet and nutrition. Every direction we look there's a different plan, theory, solution for whatever it is that ails us. It's nearly impossible to sort through it all, and all too understandable why so many people give up their power in favor of quick solutions that may indeed diminish symptoms but fail to get to the root of the problem.

As I write, the world faces a global pandemic that is challenging our health as individuals, nations, and a planet. Everything has changed. Life has moved inside— into our homes, into our hearts, into our souls. This is the perfect landscape for Sharon Holand Gelfand's G. U. T.

Method. Now, while the entire world has slowed, is the perfect opportunity to look inwards, to listen to our hearts, and to understand why and how we act, think, and make choices. Doing so provides the foundation that is essential to creating good health in our relationships—with work, play, food, movement, and most importantly, self.

I don't know that there is any such thing as a perfect diet, but I do know that the cleaner we eat, the clearer we think, the more able we are to support our good health. In my own journey, food was the conduit for change. I changed my diet and the result led me down a path to understanding and knowing my true self. Sometimes it looks like strength, empowerment, and growth, and other times, it looks messy, out-of-control, and confusing. It is a practice and a process that's never-ending. Ultimately, this approach influences how I move through the world, my connection to the earth, to community and to my physical and emotional wellbeing.

It is one thing to acknowledge that diets and trends in nutrition are likely going to change, but it's another altogether to negotiate our way through the labyrinth of options and information that falls under the scope of "wellness and nutrition." In searching, we find everything from myth and fantasy to complex science all compiled in ways that make it difficult to discern one from the other. What so many approaches casually skip over, Sharon and the G.U.T. Method provide: the acknowledgement of the unique individual as critical to understanding not only where to begin but also, how to take each step thereafter.

How do we define "normal" and "healthy" eating anyway? And how can we serve our unique constitutions without first understanding who we are and what makes us different? Doctors, friends, family, and even therapists can support our process, but only we can do the heavy lifting of listening to what is within and discovering our essential selves. This is where *The G.U.T. Method* starts. It helps us connect to the very core of our being, empowers us to let go of self-judgement and harmful messaging, and offers a much-welcome end to dieting. Sharon breaks it down and makes it doable, natural, and healthy. Finally, an approach with nothing to sell. This book is an empowering tool to help you listen, act, and live to support your good health.

The G.U.T. Method is home base—a place to check in with self, to understand nutrients rather than calories, and to start us on the path of truly being able to nourish mind, body, and soul. It is a journey of self-exploration that empowers us to take back our health. *Now* is always the best time to take inventory, redirect our focus and time, and create change and wellness in our lives. The rhythm of the entire world has changed to support us.

—*Terry Walters, bestselling author,* CLEAN FOOD

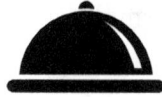

A PANDEMIC: THE ULTIMATE TEST FOR GUTS WORLDWIDE

"The human capacity for burden is like bamboo—
far more flexible than you'd ever believe at first glance."

—Jodi Picoult

Hidden in the city and stuck inside with miserable symptoms, counting on your immune system to operate properly, to fight...to fight for your life. Was that you in the spring of 2020 when a global pandemic, COVID-19, swept through our world with its fast-moving and deadly broom? Questions abound related to how well each world leader galvanized resources and handled this potentially once-in-a-lifetime crisis. As of this writing, I can tell you that we're in the thick of the devastation...particularly in New York City, where I live. Let the elected officials answer for their actions, or inaction, over the coming weeks and months. The fact that you and I are here on the same page is a good sign! I know how utterly grateful I am to be alive here with you. But I'll have questions for you throughout this healthy expedition. While being shut in and shutting down your normal life, I bet you thought a lot about life, your current state of health, relationships, purpose, and perhaps future. I hope this book helps you come to terms with those answers and sets you on the best path possible.

Instead of focusing exclusively on just one aspect of your health, we'll be talking about your gut in *every* sense of the word. This book advocates for not just your physical wellbeing, but also, for your emotional and mental wellness, and for embracing the wisdom of your insight. You know so much more than you think you do (and maybe more now, surviving a pandemic!); however, like so many women, you've been trained to mistrust self-knowledge. We've been conditioned to look to "experts" to tell us what to do: how to eat, how to exercise, how to organize our lives, how to live. The truth is that, just like Dorothy in "The Wizard of Oz," you've had the power all along. This book is going to help you get back in touch with it.

What if you had the confidence to trust yourself in a way that goes deeper than just, *how am I feeling today? Or, what diet should I go on; what supplements should I take?* In the following pages, I'll be laying out a foundation that will empower you. That will help you connect back to yourself, mind, body, and soul. That will help you feel love for yourself and joy within. That will transform your health and the way you *perceive* what being healthy means for yourself and your loved ones.

Sounds like a tall order, right? Well, I know this works because I was once in your shoes. I once stood where you are, thinking, *I did everything right. I did what I was supposed to, yet things didn't work out the way I expected. Why do I feel like something is missing? What's wrong with me? Why don't I feel alive, invigorated, vital?*

I was living a life that looked great on paper, that looked idyllic, even, from the outside: husband, kids, house. Check! I walked around like everything was great. Yet, behind closed doors, when I looked in the mirror, I didn't recognize myself. I was angry, sad, depressed, moody and unsure of myself. I was always getting sick with strep, sinus infections, IBS and debilitating migraines. On top of all these unsettling feelings, I was unhappy in my marriage, but I couldn't put my finger on why. I was shriveling up on the inside. My health was going downhill—something I didn't realize at the time because that downhill slide was made of up such small, innocuous changes. Changes that happen when you get closer to forty; at least, that's what I thought. I wondered if this was IT.

Maybe I wasn't meant for more.

Still, deep down, I kept wondering, what if…what if I was meant for more? What if everything I was taught about nutrition, health, and what makes for a happy, purpose-filled life wasn't the whole truth? What if there was something greater for me out there in the universe?

As indication of this book's manifestation, of course, I discovered that there was MORE. It didn't happen overnight but following the principles I outline in the following chapters, I learned how to live and thrive.

You may have had blinders on up until now. Most of us do, and for good reason. Big pharma and other large corporations have a stake in convincing us that there's something wrong with us that only their diets, medications, and other products can fix. Without their help, we can't possibly be okay!

That pervasive feeling of "not okay" has led us to override the wisdom of our bodies and our intuition. That feeling has disempowered us and made us doubt most, if not all, of the decisions we've made over the years. We've gotten so used to second-guessing ourselves that we've unconsciously given our power away to "experts" and people whose opinions really aren't as important as our own.

"Not okay" soon becomes "not good enough." Not a good enough daughter, mother, friend, sibling, employee, and not even a good enough dieter. Because let's face it, if we were so good at it, wouldn't we all be "skinny" and happy and healthy and have no use for all the diet books out there?

Instead, we're going on diets all the time. Keto, paleo, high protein, low fat. We follow these programs, and yet, our bodies and brains are still inflamed. It's no wonder we can't tune into ourselves and what we need. Our bodies, our engines, are all clogged and backed up like a toilet!

In order to change this downward slide, to change the conversation, we need to wake up—to secrets beyond our plates for healthier, more energetic living. To become aware of what is going on within ourselves and around us so that we can break the cycle of "not good enough." So that we can be empowered to know, to really know, that we do have the answers, that we can trust ourselves to make our own decisions based on what we need and what our bodies need, not on what someone else tells us.

You've been playing by the rules. We all have, doing what we thought we were supposed to do. Being the good wife, mother, daughter, friend, co-worker, etc. We've been doing this and thinking that everyone else is also. We've trusted that others were behaving the same way we were. We trusted advertisers to tell the truth, and doctors and pharmaceutical companies to give us medication as a last resort, when in fact, medications are often the first go-to.

What happens when we take a good look at all that, when we are willing to question the status quo? I get so excited when I think about the possibilities! When we have the right tools, when we can understand, truly understand, how to connect the dots in all areas of our lives: health, relationships with others, and relationship with self. We can then truly design our lives and find joy and purpose.

The G.U.T. Method® provides the tools you need to build the framework for your health and your life. You now have answers that you're not getting from traditional means. I've been there, standing at the empty lot. When you have the right tools in your toolbox, you'll be able to build any house you want! And the foundation is quintessential.

Here, I present your new foundation, step by step, of The G.U.T. Method®: GET connected and UNDERSTAND what's true for you and your body so that you can TAKE action and transform your health and your life.

As a global pandemic affects our lives in both real-time and unforeseen ways, it is sure to profoundly alter the world we share. In the meantime, I am honored that you may consider this guide a fundamental part of your own emergency response system for reclaiming the trajectory of your health and life.

PART I.

WHO DO YOU THINK YOU ARE, AND WHAT DO YOU KNOW?

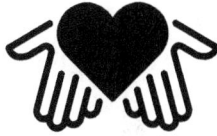

Chapter 1

FOOD IS LIKE FASHION: A HISTORY

"Simplicity is the keynote of all true elegance."

—*Coco Chanel*

I wish I had a time machine. I would travel back to 1863 to meet William Banting, an obese British undertaker who desperately wanted to lose weight. He wrote a booklet called *Letter on Corpulence, Addressed to the Public*, detailing how he lost almost fifty pounds by removing sugar and starch from his diet. I'd want to ask him how he did it. Did he listen to his body, his gut? Did he eat intuitively? After all, no one had done that before, so how did he know what to do? What happened after?

And then I'd want to curse him out for the following 150 years of diets that subsequently came along and ruined our lives! He probably didn't realize at the time what a phenomenon dieting would turn out to be in the 21st century. Some people only needed a detox to reset their bodies; others just needed to switch up their breakfast foods or drink more water throughout the day.

Then there was Dr. Jean Mayer, a French-American scientist and physiologist who would become the biggest expert on obesity in the US. He studied mice and noticed that while they all ate the same diet, the ones who weren't as active gained weight. He stated that the lack of exercise *must* be related to weight gain and so, the fitness revolution exploded. Between 1980 and 2000, memberships to fitness centers across the US more than doubled. So did the obesity rate.

I hate to admit it, but I remember those years. Jack LaLanne, Jane Fonda, and leg warmers. That was some sight. But hey, we were cool back then (although maybe the padded shoulders I wore at time may have been too much). I remember counting calories in the belief that if you restricted the number of calories you consumed and exercised more, you'd lose weight and be thin. It never worked for me, nor for friends, who were always on diets.

What we weren't taught and didn't know back then was how it wasn't about calories in, calories out, but about the food itself, the nutrients in the foods that our bodies needed. What we weren't taught was how important our gut microbiome was or how important our liver is in detoxifying our bodies and when it gets 'stopped up' we can't eliminate toxins properly. What we weren't taught was how stress, sugar and insulin are connected and that over time, too much sugar raises blood sugar levels in your body, which in turn, signals your pancreas to release insulin, shuttles the glucose in sugar out of your bloodstream and into your cells, where it is used for energy. However, excess sugar will get converted and stored as fat. What did I know about insulin back then? Or health and nutrition, for that matter? All I remember was: Diet. Count calories. Eat less. Exercise more. Take Dexatrim, so I wouldn't get hungry, and ex-lax if I ate too much. Of course, now, hindsight is 20/20 vision and I can see why I never had energy to work out and probably one of the reasons I developed IBS (irritable bowel syndrome) and other issues.

We didn't know better. Heck, I remember in college going to the local coffee shop for a bran muffin and coffee and thinking *that* was healthy because the muffin contained bran (and about a thousand calories of sugar... yeah, no wonder I couldn't lose weight).

Then in 1977, the McGovern report was released, which advocated healthier dietary goals and received a lot of pushback from the meat industry. The first dietary goals guidelines for the American public were released. The guidelines were immediately spread by TV, radio, newspapers, magazines, and healthcare providers as a road map for healthy living, and it's been a shit show ever since. Companies started creating products to help us lose weight. Advertisers created subliminal messages to us, making us believe that we needed what they had to sell. (They still do. Just look at any Facebook ad and carefully read the message.) The diet market exploded, with "experts" selling their diet foods and their amazing diets and supplements, claiming drastic results in a short period of time, including the grapefruit diet, cabbage soup diet, Slim Fast, the Master Cleanse, and countless others.

The companies and advertisers got smart. They realized that if they focused on your fears, your pain, on you not feeling pretty enough, or thin enough or tall enough, or you being so worried about everything, that you would just want to fix it quickly, then they knew they had you. They made you feel as though you are not okay. They fed you advertisements and quick fixes, keeping you hooked, instead of empowering you.

Not only were you fed advertisements; multi-billion-dollar conglomerates hired food scientists to develop products with the right amount of sugar, fat and salt to keep you addicted to buying more.

If you watched a particular ad, the slogan was, "Once you pop, you can't stop!"

According to Dr. David Kessler, in his book, *The End of Overeating*, by combining these three ingredients, our neurons are stimulated. Neurons are the basic cells of the brain. They communicate with one another and are connected via circuits. The communication can create feelings, store information and control behavior. These neurons fire off electrical signals, releasing brain chemicals, allowing them to travel to the other neurons to respond to rewarding foods. We have, in essence, become part of Pavlov's conditioning.

Then, if you look at the dietary goal guidelines, it recommends eating a certain number of calories based on your height and weight and whether you were male or female. We were taught and conditioned to count calories and if you wanted to lose weight, it was simple: Eat less!

All this messaging became imbedded in your subconscious. And with the advent of technology and social media, everything became *I must have it now*! Instant gratification. Seeing all these success stories created a need to do it also. FOMO (fear of missing out) set in. *If I don't do what they're doing, I won't get the results they're getting.* Those fears led to insecurities and in many cases, anxiety! But so many of these plans were short-term, telling you what to eat for two weeks or four weeks, without educating you. Sure, people lost weight, but what happened six months later? Many gained it back and then some. Well, that's okay because there's another diet if the first one didn't work! And the vicious cycle began. So much so that we are so disconnected from self, physically, mentally, emotionally and spiritually. We might as well be walking around in a B-rated horror flick with our heads in our hands, because we are not tuning in to self.

Food has become like fashion. Each season, there seems to be a new food or diet out there waiting to be exploited. One season, eggs are good for you. The next, they're bad. One season, coconut oil is good for you. The next, it's going to kill you. Supplements are so confusing now because no one knows who to believe or what to take. All because one expert spoke at a conference and her word became golden. What will you be able to eat this year? What will the superfood be next year?

If all these diets worked, we wouldn't have the most expensive health care system in the world, and we would certainly rate higher than No. 35 of the "healthiest nations in the world." Read the 2019 report by Bloomberg and you'll notice Spain at the top.

You Have an Internal GPS System—and Wow, It's Savvy!

Although the word "diet" dates back to the Greek word, meaning "a way of living," we have somehow twisted it into a way of thinking that makes us feel bad about ourselves, inviting us to keep looking for the magic elixir, even though there isn't one. And it's not a one-size-fits-all. We have different needs, from nutrients to emotional to physical needs, and we have to stop comparing ourselves to others.

The good news? You're not alone. The better news? There is hope! You don't have to throw in the towel and give up. You don't need to listen to or buy into those ads and messages. You don't need those new supplements or those programs telling you how to "hack" your body. All this frustration that you are feeling, the not thin enough, or smart enough, or pretty enough or good enough, is going to change. Right here. Right now.

You don't need someone to save you. You don't need to spend money on a product or an ad on Facebook that is trying to feed into that fear and keep you disconnected from your gut—your own internal GPS system.

The ads don't know you, but they do know your pain points and your fears, and they're very good at hitting those points. The people who create the ads know that if you do it, so will your friends, or vice versa. So you click on the ad, watch a video, which can take a good forty-five minutes out of your day, where they suck you in and by the end, you are just waiting to click the "buy" button or hit "subscribe and save now!" They entice you to buy their product or service, and then they tell you to join their revolution! Join their private Facebook group where you will be with like-minded people. Next, you get sucked down another rabbit hole because you read through the posts wondering what else you're missing. Now, you're addicted to the threads. Better yet, you comment on one and now you're getting notifications every time someone else comments.

Have you ever done that? Joined a group and then ended up being obsessed?

Reading the comments and then second-guessing what you thought? Maybe it's even making you anxious? You must keep checking the group because what if you are doing something wrong? What if you missed something (remember FOMO)? You went from thinking *I'll just check Facebook for five minutes,* and an hour later you're still scrolling...you're on autopilot and can't find the control to release!

The addiction continues by asking others their opinions.

The challenge with asking people their opinions is that everybody tells you what they're thinking really from only their perspective of what they know from their experience that has been right for them, not necessarily what is right for you, and you have to learn how to separate those answers and listen and feel—really feel—and tune in to when they're sharing that information with you.

Fully feel how that resonates inside of you.

Does your stomach churn, does it go nuts, or does it feel like there's a connection and there's a relief? A knowing that what they've said does feel good. When something doesn't feel good, when somebody tells us something and we're just doing it because we've asked them what they think and they're the expert, then we're not trusting ourselves. We're giving away our power and they're only giving us information from what they know.

How do they know what you need for your life experience? How do they know what you need for your lifestyle? *You know you best.* Period. No one can tell you how you are feeling, or what you are thinking, so how can they possibly know what is right for you?

This is why diets don't work. This is why when you decide to work with a practitioner, work with a nutritionist, a dietitian, a health coach or whomever, it's so important to ask them the right questions so that you find the right person to help you and what works for your lifestyle, not theirs.

This is why, when I talk to clients and we have our initial consultation, I tell them that I help them fit things into their lifestyle. I ask the right questions and help them discover the answers by uncovering their truth, by asking them enough questions that I'm reflecting to them, what they're looking for to help them come to the realization of what they need. All I've done, and all I'm doing, is being the guide, being the conduit, being the catalyst to help them feel good and trust their intuition and help them to realize that what is resonating is right for them and not for what I want or if I have an agenda.

Confession: I do have an agenda—to give you the tools to help you heal!

If you're like most of my clients, you're tired when you wake up. You don't have the same energy as you did when you were younger. Maybe you've been struggling with your weight ever since you were a kid or a teen; maybe you were teased by family and friends or felt left out. Maybe there was an emotional hole, but you were too young to articulate what that was.

You thought that dieting was the answer. If you could just lose those ten pounds, everything would be better. You'd feel great in those jeans and you thought your life would change. Maybe at first, you received a few compliments, but then after a week or so, nothing. No compliments and not only that, nothing changed in your world. Everything remained the same. Slowly, you had a snack here, dessert there, and before you knew it, the weight crept back up and you were right where you started. Maybe you thought that particular diet simply didn't work.

You went in search of another one. Maybe if you cut out sugar or fat or bread, this time would be different. Each diet, each time, you were left feeling as though you failed. *Why can't I keep this weight off?* Now: *Why am I so tired all the time?* And the fears that come up, well, you really don't want to share them with anyone because what would they think? You're tired and running out of ideas of how to get healthy. Unfortunately, it's getting worse because now you're feeling your midsection and/or hip area start to expand. You're told by your doctor, peers, friends and family that this is just how it is. "You're getting older, this is normal, so get used to it." *Really?* You wonder. *Do I have to get used to it? Is this normal? This sucks if this is all there is.*

Your joints are starting to ache in places you never expected. You may be bloated and gassy. Chalk it up to getting older? Then perimenopause hits. Your hormones are getting a little wacky. You find that you're more emotional and sensitive. You're becoming anxious. Your sex drive isn't what it used to be. Your hair is thinning and starting to fall out.

Why is this happening?

You start to feel older than your years and you want someone to fix it. You start worrying when a friend mentions a medication and wonder if maybe you have that condition because those symptoms sound *so similar* to what you are experiencing. You ask your doctor to sign over a script. You're feeling sad, and start to have bouts with depression, and are constantly apologizing for your inability to recall people's names or the things they've shared with you due to memory loss. And now, you worry if you are developing Alzheimer's. Wait...*what?*

It goes on and on spiraling out of control, yet you try so hard to keep it together and put on a good face so no one really sees your pain—if they did, you would be left standing with an open kimono, your bare soul naked with no place to hide. What if you weren't accepted for who you are? Now, you are also hiding because it's easier to stay in that pain, even though it is pain, because you just don't know what to do, and you just don't have the energy to try anymore. How long can you mask that pain with make-up, clothes, jewelry, vacations, Pilates, Barry's Boot Camp, Barre class? How can you ask for help? You're supposed to be Wonder Woman! ...Being able to juggle it all. Who will understand? Who is really listening? If you try something new, do you even have the stamina to be successful?

Holy s**t! This pain sucks. Wow, I have to admit now just re-reading these last couple of paragraphs, this sounds depressing.

I know. I totally get it. I've been there. I've purchased those products, and books and so have my clients. How many hours have I wasted? How much money flushed down the toilet on useless products, lotions and potions to turn back the clock and look for the fountain of youth?

Sometimes hundreds of dollars. Sometimes thousands of dollars.

I used to have shelves of books in my office and I'd stare at them wondering, *what am I missing? How is this possible? Why do I keep buying these books?*

The pain that you're feeling is elusive because you've just gotten so used to feeling this way that even though you may realize something is wrong and there is a better way of being, you don't consider that maybe something is missing. When something is not part of our consciousness, we have no awareness about it, which is why we keep doing the same thing over and over, expecting different results. We just get used to feeling what we're feeling and have no clue that we can feel better because we don't even know what that means.

Maybe you dread getting up and doing the same old, mundane thing, whether it's being at home with your kids, or in school or at your job. These thoughts become stories playing in your head.

Then we start talking to ourselves. Even now as you are reading this book, many of you may be thinking, "No, I don't." Case in point. If you said that, then yes, you do!

We constantly talk to ourselves and question ourselves. When it comes to our health, diets and our bodies, and so much more…the conversations are endless.

You may say to yourself how today you're going to start that diet. Today, you are not going to eat those chips in the cupboard. You go about your day and after dinner you feel proud of yourself. You did it! Almost...

You turn on the TV (or check out social media) and before you know it, you're thinking about those chips. You yell at yourself to stop thinking about them. But it doesn't stop. You think, *okay, just a few.* Before you know it, half the bag is gone, and you get pissed off wondering why you keep doing this.

Subconsciously, your mind is a tape recorder, and it keeps playing those tapes over and over despite your conscious mind telling you that you shouldn't have it. Then you get frustrated with yourself and want to give up.

Start again tomorrow?

Another self-talk scenario happens when you weigh yourself daily and are fixated with the number on the scale. Think about what that does to you. Let's say you weigh 135 and the next day it says 133. You're psyched. Wow! Don't know how that happened but great! Then the next day you weigh 136. WTF? *I didn't do anything different. How did I gain three pounds in one day?*

The vicious cycle begins. You become obsessed. We're so caught up in this loop that we drive ourselves crazy and can't let it go.

Dieting has become synonymous with breathing. We just do it.

We try to talk ourselves into changing, but it doesn't work because we haven't truly understood what that means. *Change how? Do what? And if I do change, how will that affect me, my family? My life? I've already been taught how to diet. Do I have to learn something new?* Our brains go to what is familiar, but it's not just our brain. Our gut, which has a mind of its own, is part of the equation and has another agenda.

Through my work and lessons, I've come to realize that there is so much more to being healthy than just the foods we eat. Secrets beyond the plate. I learned that I didn't know what I didn't know. I didn't know what crumbs to follow. I didn't know there was a yellow brick road that would lead to home, to me and my body.

As a matter of fact, there was so much I didn't know, because no one ever taught me or showed me the way. No one ever said, "Hey, Sharon, let's think outside the box and take a different view." Or, "Hey, Sharon, what about looking at it this way?" I thought I was all that and smarter. I definitely had a chip on my shoulder. I'm a New Yorker, for crying out loud. Don't tell me how to do things. I'll figure it out myself.

When I started my journey and realized how much I didn't know, I have to tell you, it was a little embarrassing. Then I got angry. I felt like an idiot. Like, how could I have not known this? I'm smart, how could I have not known any of this? I felt incompetent.

Maybe things aren't optimal for you. Maybe you're not where you want to be right now, but you are going to learn things and be empowered and have a shift in your health and your life. You are in control and you are okay. Your gut doesn't lie to you and you will discover in this book how to trust and understand it. With each chapter, you will be prompted with action steps so that you are learning YOU and what you need for your health and your life.

You've got this. I've got you.

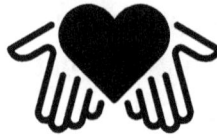

CHAPTER 2

MY GUT TALKED, I FINALLY LISTENED

"We have to dare to be ourselves, however frightening
or strange that self may prove to be."

—*May Sarton*

I grew up never questioning anything. I didn't know that
I could.

I'm a first-generation American, and my parents are
Holocaust survivors—although I didn't know that until
I was married and had children. I mean, I did know that
many members of my extended family had perished
during World War II, but not the story of what my dad and
especially, my mom, went through as children.

While this book isn't about my parents, I think it's
important to share a little of my mom's history because
it not only shaped my mom; it also shaped who I became,
or at least, who I *thought* I was supposed to be. This is
important to share because all of us, no matter where

we were born, or who raised us, or what religion we are or what our skin color is, were shaped by our past experiences, most of which started in a home.

My mom was born in 1940 in Siberia, after her parents fled Poland. While the dates aren't exactly clear, when she was around five years old, and right before the war ended, she was sent through the underground to Palestine, but she never made it there. The train she was on was diverted to Austria, where she was placed in a DP (displaced persons) camp. The camp was eventually liberated, and she was reunited with her family in Palestine (soon to become Israel). As a matter of fact, the first picture that captured her life is one with her shaved head during the time they were liberated.

I can't even imagine as a child, what that must have felt like for her, and as a parent, what that must have been like for my grandparents. Not knowing if your child is alive or dead. For my mom, not knowing if she'd ever see her parents again. The only thing she knew was that she had to survive.

Of course, now, knowing the full story, who could blame her for not sharing this story with my sister and me? I would have blocked it myself. It explains a lot about how I was raised and the belief systems I grew up with.

I was raised to work hard, do the right thing, don't ask questions, do as I was told, don't complain, don't ask for help (considered a sign of weakness—*suck it up!*), and to stop daydreaming because fantasies didn't pay the bills. There was an undercurrent of fear, but of course, back then, I wasn't aware of it. Life was about being practical, strong, resilient, and independent, and most of all, surviving.

How my mom's story and my childhood played out for me was that I wanted to please my parents, so as a child and throughout my adolescence, I tried to do what they wanted. The more I tried to please them, however, the more resentful I became. I could never really articulate why I was always angry, especially at my mom, but looking back now, it seemed that anytime I would say something, or ask for something, I was met with resistance.

Then there were times when I was just simply afraid to ask for anything because the answer was always no. "Mom, can I sleep over at Lisa's house?" *No.* "Why?" *Because I said so.* "Mom, can she sleep here?" *No.* "Why?" *You see her every day at school. I don't see a reason to have a sleepover.*

I would get so angry sometimes that I would run upstairs and slam my door (I mean, really slam it, like a 6.7 on the Richter scale). I realized that I didn't truly possess a voice to say anything, so I stopped trying; instead, I became rebellious. What could I get away with without her knowing? Remember, I had no idea how traumatic my mother's childhood had been, and I was a typical rebellious tween/teen.

I remember a few summers that we spent up in the Catskills, at a bungalow colony. If you watch "The

Marvelous Mrs. Maisel", you'll basically see my summers in the 70s, at Pancrest Lodge in South Fallsburg. I have to digress and share that in the series, Midge Maisel takes her measurements every day, and not just her waist or bust or thighs, but each shin, calf, arm and wrist. Guess what? So does her mother! Did her mother teach her this or did she just observe it long enough to think that this is what she should do also?

I remember when I was a teenager, I would watch my mom put on makeup every Saturday evening before she and my dad went out. I would watch her apply eye shadow, mascara, crème rouge and lipstick, and when she left for the evening, I would go into her vanity drawer and take out all of her makeup and try it on, pretending I, too, was going out.

I also remember that at every meal we had together as a family, my mom would not permit us leave the kitchen table until we finished everything on our plate. *Do you know how many starving kids there are in the world? You're lucky to have this food!* Even if we were full, we had to finish our food. (I didn't have a dog to feed it to under the table like you see in the movies.) I would sometimes feel so nauseous and fat and would take ex-lax to get rid of the food since the idea of putting my finger down my throat to expel the food grossed me out. Now, of course, looking back, it's easy to have 20/20 vision and see how some of my dysmorphia developed.

Diary of Diets...and Other Great Escapes

Pretending. Watching. Copying. Our mothers. Fathers. Older siblings? Is that where you get your beliefs from? Watching and emulating? Wanting to be like your parents? Or the opposite? Not liking what you saw and knowing you didn't want that in your life and rebelling.

Getting back to rebelling and the Catskills, my friends and I would walk into town to the corner to Poppins Diner. We'd eat and then flush the bill down the toilet and sneak out the back door, or go across the street to the local five and dime to see who could take the most expensive item without paying (I cringe when I think that I stole anything!). The worst I could do was sneak an *Archie* comic book under my shirt. Yeah, we're talking that kind of rebellion. Sacrilege to some, nothing compared to other types of rebellion. Don't judge! For me, I was just trying to fit in and feel a part of something.

This behavior was a Band-Aid. Escape mechanisms. I swallowed my emotions and feelings, especially anger. From an early age, I suffered from stomachaches, and from constipation to diarrhea, then back to constipation. I frequently got sties, and my eyes were usually inflamed. I was embarrassed to be seen because my eyes were so red.

By the time I got my period, oh boy, was I moody. I had terrible cramps and heavy periods. I didn't want to go to school because I felt miserable, but staying home was not an option.

You know what happened when puberty hit. My body changed in ways I couldn't control. What did I do next? I started dieting. Dexatrim pills and the grapefruit diet to start and then, as the years went on, every diet I could get my hands on. I thought that maybe, just maybe, if I could control what I ate and how much I weighed, I'd be happy. The problem with dieting though, as you've undoubtedly experienced, is that diets don't work long-term. I'd lose weight, my pants would feel big, and I'd be happy for a minute. But nothing seemed to change in my life. It all stayed the same. To be honest, I wasn't sure what I was looking for, but I kept expecting that losing the weight and being "thin" would fulfill something. I didn't have the words then to describe what that something was. My world stayed the same and soon enough, the weight would creep back on. I would go on this yo-yo dieting journey for years, leading me to a host of other health complaints like hypoglycemia and irritable bowel syndrome. I had become a creature of habit. The dieting habit. There *had* to be one, just one diet that would do it.

I didn't realize that I was barely surviving. At a time without the Internet. I had encyclopedias and the library, but I couldn't find what I was looking for. I had no way of understanding that my body was sending me signals, symptoms that were never bad enough to send me to the hospital, thank god! I remember when my mother did take me to the doctor, he told me to take Metamucil for constipation. My mom didn't help the situation because when I complained that I felt fat or my stomach hurt, I didn't feel any encouragement. She never felt what I was feeling and would say so, and then add: *You'll be fine.* But I wasn't fine, and it was so frustrating and embarrassing.

Don't get me wrong. I know now that my mom did the best that she could with the tools she had, but I was a kid who just wanted to make her parents happy. While I didn't consciously know it at the time, I used food and dieting to try and find some control in my life, and for emotional comfort, because when I went clothes shopping with my mother, it felt like I was naked on a runway being judged with every piece of clothing I put on. *Nothing ever fit.* My mother would choose clothes that I didn't like, and I would get angry. My mother didn't have much patience back then and would get annoyed and either not buy anything or buy what she wanted for me, and that was that. No questions asked. Regardless, I always looked for ways to please my parents.

I happened to be good with numbers (at least, back then I was), so I went into banking and finance and became a commercial banker; very respectable for a first-generation American! At least there, I could hide behind the numbers and maintain control of my life.

Everything is black and white to a banker. After all, numbers are numbers. One plus one will always equal two. I lived my life that way for a long time. Since everything was always linear, so were my expectations and assumptions.

By the time I got married and had kids, I thought my life was under control, yet I became hypoglycemic, anemic, had chronic migraines, eczema, mood swings, IBS...oh, and a pituitary adenoma (a benign brain tumor in the pituitary) that messed up my hormones. But I was too busy with life, too busy continuing to live the life that I was taught to live and not question. To live a life where I got a good job that paid well, married someone of the same religion who could support and care for a family, save money, and be financially secure. Very traditional. *Be the good mother, the good wife, the good everything.*

Deep down, I felt that something just wasn't right. I couldn't put my finger on it and it was making me uncomfortable. I showed up as someone I didn't recognize (imposter syndrome), trying harder and harder to fit in, to make things right; and I felt shame and embarrassment. Something wasn't aligned. I had become disconnected from my body and didn't realize that my body was sending me signals and I was ignoring them. One doctor prescribed a cream for the eczema. Another one prescribed shots for my migraines. Another one put me on a different medication for my IBS. I was even put on anti-depressants a few months before my oldest son had his bar mitzvah (and then took myself off of them because it felt like I was just putting a Band-Aid on a wound that needed stitches).

Yet, I considered myself healthy; after all, the doctors never indicated that I wasn't. I had compartmentalized everything because it was easier to be in denial, so I could just stay on my path and survive another day.

I was stuck on the treadmill of life, though I didn't consciously realize it because this was how I was raised, and I thought that there was nothing I could do. I found myself shrinking and feeling smaller; my world and my walls started to close in around me.

A Diagnosis and a Turning Point

In 2007, when I heard my 12-year-old son turn white and ask me, "Am I going to die?" I felt as though someone had shoved their hand into my body and pulled my heart out, leaving me gasping for air. We were sitting in the doctor's office, where he had just been diagnosed with Crohn's, ulcerative colitis, and ileitis, all part of irritable bowel disease (IBD). I had never heard the term before.

I took a deep breath. "You're going to be fine," I told him.

I hugged him tightly, but my stomach was in knots as I watched him trying to process the word "disease". I knew nothing about Crohn's. I did what any other parent would do: I asked Dr. Google. Five hours later, 100 tabs open, and I had a splitting headache. I was so confused. There was so much information and so much fear. I didn't know what to believe, who to listen to or where to even start.

What I did notice was that so much pointed to the gut, food, supplements, and lifestyle, that I couldn't ignore it. The more that I learned, the more the banker in me started to analyze everything. I had more questions than answers and this time, I was not going to sit back and allow myself to not be heard. This time, I was going to be speak up and advocate for my son and my family.

I decided to go to grad school to get a master's in clinical nutrition and later, get certified as a functional nutritionist, all so that I could help my son. Oh, and I decided to undertake this while going through a divorce, with kids in high school and college and with a heap of hormones raging in my house.

What I discovered was that this was just the beginning of the journey. What I discovered was that there had always been signs, a trail of breadcrumbs to guide me in the right direction but I hadn't seen them. I was too busy being in my head and so disconnected from my body. You know, people say that the universe sends you signs over and over for you to pay attention to. You could say it's unfortunate that the signs came in the form of my son's diagnosis. But I look at it as a blessing in disguise. That my own health issues were so compartmentalized that I would not have done anything about it because I was too busy taking care of everyone else.

When it came to taking care of my son and springing to action, I wouldn't change any aspect of my journey. I could easily have played victim and thought the "what if" I had listened to my body back then? What if I had realized back when I was in the hospital for a day of X-rays, MRIs and CAT scans to see why I couldn't move my neck, thinking I was paralyzed, that it was a pinched nerve as a result of years of stress accumulating in my neck? The universe had sent signs, jolts to my body, to wake the hell up. I could have easily gone down the rabbit hole of wondering if I could have avoided Zach's diagnosis. In pure transparency,

I did at first, feel guilt that I had somehow been the reason. But I chose to shift my perspective and realize that I don't know what I would have done. I guess I hadn't wanted to see anything that could have been contrary to what I thought my life should look like because I was protecting my ego.

It was part of my journey to learn what I needed to, to understand what I needed to, in order to take the path, I was meant to. And that is true for you, too.

The saying, "The teacher appears when the student is ready," is true for everyone. Some people are ready sooner, some later, some never. It's not about right or wrong. It's about being where you are. It's about shifting your perspective and putting your ego on the side to give you the space to allow new information to enter.

If you could sit still for a few minutes and breathe in and out, asking yourself, "What do I need to know?" you will hear a voice in your head that may give you an answer. Here, accept talking to yourself until it sets in that this is your intuition, in your own voice, and with wisdom to guide you.

This book is here to help you get back to basics for your own life. Your health. Your relationships: with yourself and those you surround yourself with. It's taking a look at your house and owning that there are cracks in the foundation and the walls. Owning that if you keep avoiding the work that needs to be done, that it will have a ripple effect that will be more costly in the long run. You can be proactive or reactive. It's your choice. Only you can decide.

I think the biggest misconception we have is that we made mistakes that we can't recover from. But really, are they mistakes? Everything is about choices. You don't look at a situation and ask yourself if you should make the mistake! You contemplate choices. Yet, when things don't work out in our favor, we go to the negative. It's no surprise that we react. That's how society and our parents and ancestors taught us. You made a mistake, shame on you! Imagine yelling at a toddler for falling while learning to walk. We would never do that. They're learning and they keep trying until they get it and we keep clapping, always offering them encouragement.

That's how I encourage you to look at your health and your life. As you continue throughout this book, you may experience epiphanies that will help you see the path you've taken that has led you up to this point.

When I think back to my journey and how my life played out, I made a shift in my perspective and realized I needed to learn so that I could teach others. I was given a gift. I needed to experience every pain, every moment of joy, sadness, laughter and crying so that I could grow and help others do the same. At the end of the day, the one thing I will never regret is getting married or getting divorced. I wouldn't have my amazing children without that marriage. I wouldn't have been able to grow and provide the space for my kids to do the same if I hadn't gotten divorced because I would have suffocated as well as my kids. My life is fuller, richer and brighter because of them.

Whatever choice you made, while it may not have worked out in your favor, perhaps there was a reason and you learned something from it. It's okay. You're okay.

As you continue through this book, you'll discover that all that you've gone through, all the dots, are now ready to be connected.

WRITING EXERCISE
DIGEST AND DISCOVER

Take a few minutes to think about your own journey. Did you have moments when your gut told you to go in one direction, but you chose another? Did you have moments when you kept getting signs to take action on an issue and you listened? Or didn't? Maybe you keep eating a food that you know gives you gas or a stomachache or some other symptom, but you decide to take an antacid because you don't want to give up that food (even if it doesn't serve you). Take time to reflect without judging yourself. Give yourself space to be the observer of what is going on.

Write it down.

_____

_____

_____

_____

_____

_____

_____

_____

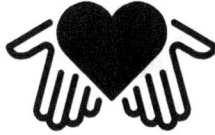

CHAPTER 3

YOU HAVE CHOICES— CHANGE THE TAPES OF YOUR SUBCONSCIOUS

....

"The truth does not change according to our ability
to stomach it."

—*Flannery O'Connor*

....

Common side effects include nausea, vomiting and diarrhea. Don't worry. There's another medication to help you with the side effects of the first medication.

Wait...what? Why are we listening to all the ads on TV and not to ourselves? When did we stop trusting our gut?

We have been looking at health and nutrition completely wrong. We have been taught and conditioned to focus on counting calories, diet, exercise, get eight hours of sleep, and to expect our bodies to fall apart as we age.

We've been hearing these messages over and over, every day of every week of every year, our whole lives.

It's been passed down to us from generation to generation and reinforced by marketing and advertising, so much so, that these instructions have become unconscious. The information is so ingrained in us that we believe it as fact and so it becomes our truth. Notice, in the ads telling you that you can do more to lower your blood sugar because your body can still make its own insulin (but take this medication to activate your body to release it), everyone is smiling and the music makes you feel good. They're even calm when they talk about the possible side effects of "stroke and death" as though it's no big deal!

What Pain? What Pill?

In the movie, "The Matrix", Morpheus explains to Neo that he is living in the Matrix. This is the world that has been pulled over your eyes to blind you from the truth.

It's all around you. Even in the very room you are sitting in right now reading this book. But no one can be told what it is. You have to see it and feel it for yourself.

Morpheus offers Neo a choice of two realities. Take the blue pill. The story ends. You wake up in your bed and believe what you want to believe. *Or* take the red pill, stay in Wonderland, and see how you can grow.

We live in two realities, one in which we are being fed marketing messages and believing what experts are telling us to believe. Our second reality is owning our ability to wake up and take our power back, listening to our bodies and being our own health experts. In this book,

I'm going to help you redefine what that means to you and your health.

Total Nourishment

People have defined *health* as being free from illness or injury and nutrition as eating foods to give us energy and to grow. In reality, health encompasses so much more than counting calories or exercise or sleep. Being healthy is about *nourishment.* Nourishment from our relationships with our family, friends, and co-workers. Nourishment from our mindset, managing our stress levels, developing the ability to connect to our own souls and self-care, and from our belief systems—knowing what our truth is. Nourishment so that we can pull the leaves of the artichoke and get to the best part...the heart.

In order to uncover the health spectrum for yourself, you must first be open to the idea that you don't know what you don't know.

Noel Burch developed the Conscious Competence Ladder in the 1970s. The ladder helps us understand our thoughts and emotions as we learn new skills. While this model was built for people in business, it can be applied to all areas of our lives, including relationships, including our relationship with food.

The four levels are:

Unconscious Incompetence:
I don't know what I don't know. "Dieting is the answer to

losing weight and being healthy. Keep trying diets until you find the right one."

Conscious Incompetence:

I know that I don't know. This is where we start to develop consciousness and realize that hey, those diets didn't work, and start to have hope but quickly self-sabotage because of the realized failure of what didn't work before. Here, you see yourself in the mirror and realize you are doing it wrong. You try to undertake measures to change but are unsure really of what path to take and this is where most people quit because they get frustrated. They don't realize that while they are trying different diets, they're still diets, so they're doing the same thing over and over, expecting different results.

Consciously Competent:

I grow and know and it starts to show. Here, you are dedicating yourself to improving in all aspects (i.e. eating healthy and incorporating lifestyle shifts). Here, you are creating the space to observe and become aware of your actions without judgment. You start getting excited realizing that there's a new way to be and if that is true, what else is out there for you to learn?

Unconsciously Competent:

I simply continue because of what I know. You may be intrigued by the Facebook ads but no longer feel that you are missing the fountain of youth if you don't click on the ad. You're no longer being sold to and are free from the external mind chatter and noise because you are tapped in to your soul and inner guidance system: your savvy GPS.

I must note that Burch's Conscious Competence Ladder is similar to another favorite example, in Portia Nelson's *There's a Hole in My Sidewalk*. It goes like this:

"Chapter One of My Life. I walk down the street. There's a deep hole in the sidewalk. I fall in. I am lost. I am helpless. It isn't my fault. It still takes forever to find a way out.

Chapter Two. I walk down the same street. There's a deep hole in the sidewalk. I pretend I don't see it. I fall in again. I can't believe I'm in the same place! But it isn't my fault. And it still takes a long time to get out.

Chapter Three. I walk down the same street. There's a deep hole in the sidewalk. I see it there. I still fall in. It's a habit! My eyes are open. I know where I am. It is my fault. I get out immediately.

Chapter Four. I walk down the same street. There's a deep hole in the sidewalk. I walk around it.

Chapter Five. I walk down a different street."

[Reprinted with permission.]

How many times do we walk down the same path with our eyes closed? That was me. As I mentioned earlier when I shared my story about my son, I was asleep. I didn't get any of this until my son was diagnosed with Crohn's, and I wanted answers. I started to worry about his health. I asked if there was anything I should change in his diet (somehow, something inside of me knew there must be a connection), but I was told not to worry because the medicine was all he needed. I didn't know what to do, so I listened to the professional. A week later, when my son started complaining that he was getting worse and that it was the medicine, I called his doctor, who insisted that it was the disease and to stay on the medicine.

You know, when you're a kid, everything in life is a possibility. You're not jaded by society. You live freely in your naiveté, and many of us lose that, as we get older. Not my son. He didn't care what the doctor said, and he wouldn't take no for an answer. He was listening to his body—his gut—and insisted that it was the medicine.

I heard a voice in me shouting, "What are you doing? Why aren't you listening to your son? Why? Because he's a kid?"

So, thankfully, I did because he was right. It was the medicine. This created a crack in my existing belief system. It made me question what else I was missing that I needed to know to help my son heal, and also, my own health and whether what I was doing was the right thing for me. (Now, I see the hole, but I'm still not walking down a different street.)

I thought I was healthy. I was exercising, eating right; however, I was also taking:

- Imitrex shots for migraines

- Parlodel for pituitary adenoma

- Antibiotics for chronic sinus and strep infections

- Creams for eczema

- Antacids for IBS

- Iron for anemia

- ...and eating frequently for hypoglycemia

I never questioned any of it. I was healthy. But I was also so tired. I had no energy. I was cranky. I figured it must be that I was getting older. Or that I needed "that pill" they talked about in the ad.

I lived in this altered reality until my son's diagnosis woke me up. That wake-up call helped me get rid of the medications and heal my own body as I helped my son to heal his. (Now, I'm ready to walk down a different street and avoid the hole!)

Spoiler alert: Neo dies at the end of "The Matrix" ... or so we think. Trinity is with his body and says, "Get up." For those who haven't seen the movie, Trinity is a computer programmer and hacker who has escaped the matrix and who has fallen in love with Neo. Neo opens his eyes, stands up, looks at the agents as they start shooting at him, puts his hand out, and says, *"No."* The bullets stop in midair and drop to the floor.

Neo is not playing the game anymore. He's chosen his new reality. You can, too. Read that sentence again. You can, too. I sometimes think that we don't realize that we actually have choices. We're *reacting* to situations, instead of hitting the pause button, and then choosing to be proactive.

For instance, your boss asks you to stay late to finish a project. It has to be done and it's your job. However, you have plans to meet friends for a birthday celebration dinner. You can't go to the birthday celebration dinner, you tell your friends, because *you have no choice*. You have to stay and do your job. You did choose though. You chose your job over the birthday celebration. You chose unconsciously. You weren't aware. And this isn't about judgment. It's just an observation of how we make choices but aren't always aware that we are doing so.

Or, let's say you are going away on vacation. You feel like you have to diet and starve yourself before your trip and lose weight because you just know you will gain weight on that trip. Your mindset is fixed because of past experiences. You think you have no choice. That you have to go on a diet, or you'll be stressed out the whole trip and have to diet when you get home. There is always a choice, however.

Once you realize that it's not all black and white, the world starts to shift. Your view starts to shift, and new possibilities appear, and you start to get excited, wondering, wow, what if I don't diet before I leave but instead, I really tune in to my body and eat nutrient-dense food. Then when I go on vacation, I enjoy the foods, but I think consciously about what I am eating and I learn to eat intuitively for what my body needs, while also indulging in a few desserts and a glass (or two or a bottle) of wine.

If I shift my perspective, I am making a conscious choice to enjoy life! I just did that recently in Italy. My sister and I had an amazing trip to Umbria. Some sister bonding time and a spiritual retreat attached at the end. We knew we'd be drinking lots of wine and eating lots of pasta. We didn't gain one pound and I didn't get one headache drinking the wine. Now, at home, I can't really drink red wine because the sulfites give me a nasty headache the next day. But Italy makes wine differently and I was fine. The way they make pasta is also different than in the states because their food supply is different. So, I enjoyed without pigging out. I made a choice.

Imagine if I chose not to have the wine or the pasta. Imagine if I hadn't shifted my perspective. First, I'd be missing out on amazing food and grapes and worrying about gaining weight and the diet I would have to go on when I returned. Second, I might as well have stayed home. With continued practice on awareness of life and what I stressed over, I realized I was wasting time with fear instead of joy and excitement. This trip was about all the joy and wonder of the experience and without fear of that nasty four-letter word, "diet".

By shifting your perspective and actively choosing, you start to get excited about other possibilities of what you can do. It's your life. Only you can know what you need.

And it's not about agenda. It's not about forcing you to fit a cookie cutter mold. It's not telling you to go to the USDA chart. It's not telling you to go to myplate. gov. It's telling you to listen intuitively to yourself. Listen intuitively to your gut, to your soul, to that voice inside so that you understand you what you need. If you don't understand and you don't get connected, it's really hard to take action because it gets so overwhelming, which is why you have to chunk it down, which is why The G.U.T. Method® was created. To chunk it down, so that you can get connected to all parts of your being and to give yourself time to do it. To say, for example, that this week I'm going to focus on connecting to symptoms. I'm going to focus on writing down how I'm feeling after I eat.

You need a manual for your body (much like the manual for your car), that will break it down, simplify it so that it fits you. So that it fits *your* lifestyle because someone else's "diet" book is not the answer. Counting calories or starving yourself is not the answer. You know that if it were the answer, you would be where you want to be. Your body, your health, would be there, at the finish line. You think you're doing everything right, but you may wake up one day with a diagnosis and wonder, *how did I get here?*

The G.U.T. Method® in Action, with Your Participation

This manual was designed to help you discover what you need to thrive and be healthy. It's filled with sections to journal in. There is plenty of space for you to read, learn and write it down so that you can keep track of your progress: **Digest and Discover**. Sit with your thoughts and listen to your inner wisdom. Wisdom is innate. It needs help getting stronger, like your muscles. The more you work out, the stronger you feel. The more you practice the steps, the stronger your mind will feel to be able to trust itself; you will trust your decisions, feel great, decrease stress, get healthy and lose weight (*if* that's what you need). This is your guide to help you shift from your unconscious to your conscious, to help you change the tapes of the subconscious, to help you get connected to you, your body, and your mind so that you can understand what it all means to you and your lifestyle. You can then take action, trust yourself, tune in to your intuition, and transform your life to the one you were meant to live. Part II of this book will break down each component and give you tools so that you can create your blueprint—one that is on your terms, one that understands that what you need comes from within you.

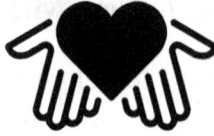

CHAPTER 4

YOUR TWO BRAINS

"The definition of insanity is doing the same thing over and over again but expecting different results."

—*Albert Einstein (presumably)*

Trust your gut.

When you hear this, what comes to mind? Does it bring up thoughts about intuition? That unspoken sense that invisibly guides you, notifying you that something's up? Does it have you question authority versus trusting yourself?

What if trusting your gut went deeper? Literally, into the core of your being?

Your gut is a magical place. Trillions of helpful bacteria live there, sending signals to other parts of your body. Some scientists refer to our gut as our *second brain*; some even go so far as to call it our real brain.

Your gut tells you when it's hungry, and when you've eaten too much. You feel butterflies in your stomach when you're in love. It may feel like moths are flying around inside when you're nervous (no disrespect meant to moths).

How about when you're stressed and maybe at times that you're not able to express yourself? A lot of that stress can get swallowed up and can turn into anxiety, and manifest physically creating inflammation in your gut and your brain! Your body may over-produce stomach acid, which could lead to acid reflux, heartburn, a sour stomach, a headache, even a migraine.

This could lead to OTC (over-the-counter) medications, which just puts a Band-Aid on the problem and doesn't address the root cause. Taken on a long-term basis (even when the stress goes away) the medications inhibit the creation of the good bacteria that we want. This throws off the balance of bacteria in our gut and can throw off our body's ability to tune in, listen and *trust* what it is telling us.

It can inhibit our body's ability to produce enough serotonin, the "feel good" neurotransmitter. Serotonin sends signals between our nerve cells and if the body is not producing enough, the signals that help us feel all the good are stunted. When that happens, it can lead to crankiness and lashing out, especially to those closest to us.

I remember before Zach was diagnosed, he would get moody. At first, I chalked it up to the fact that his dad and I were getting divorced and to an 11-year-old, that is not one of those life events that you want to remember. Even though we worked on making our parting as amicable as possible, change to a child is scary. Children want and need stability. Heck, I was scared, too. I couldn't even imagine what my kids were feeling. Each of them handled the situation differently, so to the other two, their brother was looking for attention. He was also in the throes of the tween years, which are awkward enough, so I didn't think much of it. Until he was diagnosed.

That's putting it mildly. I really didn't even realize the connection until I started grad school and started putting the pieces together, looking back at the timeline of events. I had journaled about some of the circumstances but being in the midst of a life-altering event, I was just doing my best trying to keep my head above water (and self-medicating with wine every night!). Plus, Zach was able to tell me that the medication was making his symptoms worse, why would I even think that his behavior could be a symptom of his condition also? How many symptoms could he possibly have? Of course, now, with the awareness and knowledge I have, looking back, it is crystal clear how his emotional and physical self was so intertwined!

What I noticed was that as he started to heal, his behavior started to change. Yes, he was still acting out and trying to get attention, but his *explosive* behavior started to slow down. His eczema went away, his allergies were getting better and his gut was starting to heal. While he did need medicine, making small shifts in food choices, adding in supplements and shifting lifestyle habits created so much more balance in his life.

What if bringing back those magical connections from your gut could be made via some simple changes for you? You don't have to have a diagnosis to understand that your gut is key. How great would it be if you could get back to feeling like your old self? Do you remember what that feels like?

Reviews of studies published in the journal, *General Psychiatry*, suggests, "people who experience anxiety symptoms might be helped by taking steps to regulate the microorganisms in their gut using probiotic and non-probiotic food and supplements." (More on this later.)

Coming back to the way your body and gut brain were meant to connect, I'll let you in on a secret: It is the most important section of this book and your life. I'm not being flippant here. I know that sounds so dramatic, but I can tell you, from my own life experience, my family, and from my clients, those aha moments, those epiphanies you'll have, the bridge of going from unconscious to conscious, wow! Those moments that created your belief systems, and that moment when you get it, when you become so aware, so attune, your heart will feel like it is going to explode with everything amazing. *You deserve this.* You deserve to live your best life now and you only have one life in this body. Isn't it time to give it the love and nurturing it needs so it can give you the energy, love and light that you deserve? Yes, yes, and yes!

The World Health Organization (WHO) defines health as physical, mental, and social wellbeing, and as a resource for living a full life. It refers not only to the absence of disease, but also, the ability to recover and bounce back from illness and other problems.

"Health" has gotten rather complicated though. We're not bouncing back from stress and illness. We think we are doing everything right, but our bodies are falling apart. There's a crack in the system, and we need to start paying attention. And to what? No one is telling us how, and we're developing chronic conditions that affect the way we live and the length of our lifespans.

Autoimmune disease, where our immune system mistakenly attacks itself, is now recognized as a major health crisis in the US. The National Institutes of Health (NIH) has stated that there are over 80 different types of autoimmune diseases, including rheumatoid arthritis, lupus, MS and Hashimoto's. Thirty years ago, about one in 400 people developed an autoimmune disease. Today, one in 12 Americans, and one in 9 women, have an autoimmune disease. That's astounding! One in 9.

What about diabetes? More than 30 million Americans have diabetes. As of 2017, asserts American Diabetes Association, this cost America $357 billion a year. This includes $237 billion in direct medical costs and $90 billion in reduced productivity. The striking part is that Type 2 diabetes is getting diagnosed younger and younger. Before the obesity epidemic in the US, Type 2 diabetes was practically unheard of in people under 30. It is no longer uncommon for children to be diagnosed with this condition.

How did we get here? How did *you* get here?

I'll admit that's a loaded question because it goes deeper than just the food we eat.

We have to pay attention to so much more than our parents and grandparents had to pay attention to. We must consider what chemicals in the environment, metals like mercury, aluminum and arsenic, as well as cleaning and skin care products, may be doing to our bodies; how it's affecting our gut, our brain, the correlation between the two, and the increase in all these medical conditions that are being diagnosed annually. It's enough to give anyone a headache, especially when we are bombarded with information on a daily basis.

At the beginning of the book, I mentioned how we need to wake up and become aware of what is going on within ourselves and around us so that we can break the cycle and stop passing down all the crap to our kids and future generations.

It's time to start asking yourself questions. What you are putting into your mouth? Is it food grown from the earth? From an animal or the ocean? Is it coming from a factory, delivered to the store in a box that sits on a shelf for six months but has a claim on the front that sounds enticing? If it is sitting on a shelf and not decomposing, what is it doing in your body? And we have to wonder what the pesticides being used are doing to our health. Pictures of workers in Hazmat suits and gas masks spraying fields. If they were safe, why all that protection? In 2019, Monsanto pleaded guilty to the spraying of a banned pesticide in Hawaii. What's next?

It means looking at the products you are putting on your skin and the products you use to clean your house (and for those who work in offices, what cleaning products are being used there).

When I moved back to the city, I started to notice that I was getting slight headaches. I started writing down when I would get them and realized they would occur around the same time the maintenance staff would vacuum the hallway. There was a smell in the hallway on my floor when they were vacuuming. It took a few weeks for me to make the connection that they were spraying chemicals on the carpet to clean them and the smell was seeping under my door and into my apartment and giving me a headache. WHAT? Crazy! But that's how sensitive I was. So, I went down to the office, spoke to the building manager and the staff taking care of the vacuuming, and while they still use that cleaner, they don't use it on the stretch of hallway to my apartment (fortunately I am in an end unit).

These are those seemingly innocuous moments that add up over time. We can't escape it completely unless you want to live in the woods and eat bamboo shoots and leaves, but you can do your best to control what you can control and let go of what you can't control.

Health also means asking yourself what you are putting in your mind. Are you minding your thoughts? This includes self-talk. The self-sabotage. We need to start thriving instead of just surviving.

Before you even figure out where to start, I want you to first commit to tuning out the noise for now, so that you can learn more about yourself and what *you* need. Commit to not clicking on the ads for the next best pill solution. Commit to not Googling the experts you may have been following and, I'd even take it a step further and say, unsubscribe (*for now*) to any newsletters that you may be getting that are health- and wellness-related (or anything that will take you to external reading material that will invariably confuse you even further and waste precious time). Commit to not going on a diet! There is no diet on this planet that will work for everyone because you are each unique. You may have the same organs in your body, but your biochemistry is completely unique; therefore, the nutrients you need will be different than that of your friend, sister, mother, father, etc. *Period.*

I can feel your eyes boring into me right now, through these pages. Hear me out. During this writing, I spoke at a few companies about stress and anxiety and how it affects your body, productivity and relationships. During the Q & A, someone asked me: "Sharon, what do you think about Dr. Gundry's *Plant Paradox* and Dave Asprey's *Bulletproof* diet? Should I read and follow what they're saying? It's so confusing because there is too much to do, and supplements to buy there and elsewhere on the Internet."

I was thrilled to get this question. I smiled, looked at the audience and said, "Before you start searching externally for the answer, let's start within. Start with you and understand you first. Because once you can do that, you'll then know and understand where to go next. You'll learn to trust yourself (which we'll discuss more in the next section of the three-step method) and then you'll know which external sources are the right ones for you."

To me, this, in a nutshell, is what will help you avoid chasing the next best pill or diet. This understanding of you has to start from within. Not a doctor, nutritionist, acupuncturist, naturopath, chiropractor because they (or I) don't know exactly what you are feeling. We can ask questions and help you connect the dots, but if you don't share all the information or the right questions aren't asked, there will be gaps—which is why you have to learn the nuances of your body's signals. Once you can articulate and keep track of where you were then and where you are now, then the path will become clear. You will be filled with possibilities for the healthiest life that you didn't even know existed.

WRITING EXERCISE
HEALTH COMMITMENT: SIGN AND COMMIT

Read the statement below and sign and agree to make this commitment to yourself:

I,

———————————————————————————————

commit to learning first about myself; to using this three-step G.U.T. Method™ to get connected, become aware, understand, tune in, trust myself to take action and transform my life.

I commit to unsubscribing from e-mails that drive me crazy. I commit to not clicking on Facebook ads that are trying to sell me the next best diet, supplement or plan because it sounds great and the comments make it feel like this is going to be my solution.

I commit to not spending unnecessary money on supplements or programs because they sound great.

I commit to stop eating advertisements and instead tune in to me and learn what nourishes me.

I commit to not buying the next new product at the grocery store because it says it will give me energy, grow god knows what on my body, or it's on sale.

I commit to honoring my body, my temple, and becoming proactive about my health.

I commit to being empowered so that my biggest asset gives me the energy, strength, space and love so that I can be grounded in my core beliefs and be lifted to help others.

I commit to being open and believing in the possibilities of health, love and life.

From this day forward, I commit to me because if I don't put the oxygen mask on myself first, I will be in no shape to be of assistance to others.

(Sign your name)

I'm so glad we got that out of the way! Now, we can focus on where to start. It can feel daunting and overwhelming, but like cleaning out your house, you start by picking one room at a time. In this case, we start with a foundation of what your symptoms are, how long you've been feeling them and how it is affecting your life. This isn't about judgment or beating yourself up over what didn't work in the past. Everything will unfold as you go through the process and by being kind to yourself during this time. We are going to wipe the slate clean and just start from here. This point. Today.

As I was saying earlier, the challenge we are all faced with is wondering how we got here and what we should do. We are trying to do everything at once and so get nothing done. Because our brain cells are on fire all the time, because we are getting bombarded with so many messages, we don't take a moment to ask ourselves what we need. We don't take the time to listen to what our intuitive self needs.

One of my clients, Suzy, was obsessed with Facebook ads. Looking at Suzy was like looking at a magazine picture. From the outside, she looked like she had it all. She's petite, beautiful, and in great shape. She has a loving husband and kids, and a job she really enjoys. To boot, she is gluten- and dairy-free and eats whole foods. Now, you know there's a "but" coming. Suzy's insides were falling apart due to IBS, aching joints, and shoulder surgery. She had previously been treated by her doctor with antibiotics for small intestinal bacterial overgrowth (SIBO).

Suzy came to me after going to different practitioners, spending thousands of dollars, and still not feeling well. She was understandably frustrated that no one was able to figure out what was going on and thought that this was what happened when you get older. After having her complete a stool test and getting the results (along with her intake form), Suzy went on a simple nutrition and supplement/botanical protocol and tweaked some of the snacks she was eating. She couldn't believe how much better she felt.

Here's the kicker. Suzy had filled out the symptoms questionnaire I gave her, but never indicated that she suffered from a runny nose and eczema around that area. It took her husband remarking that she was "no longer carrying a box of tissues everywhere" for her to realize that she had been living with the sniffles for over twenty years, not knowing that they were signals from her body that something was off. She was so used to feeling that way that she never thought about it. As far as she was concerned, having a runny nose was her "normal"—so much so that she didn't even note it on the questionnaire. She was disconnected from her body's symptoms. Her runny nose was a blind spot.

What blind spots might you have? What signals might your body be sending that you're missing?

Once Suzy got in touch with her body (and with her husband's help) and connected to what it was telling her, she began to be aware of signals like that runny nose. You would think that the story ends there, but of course it doesn't. You see, Suzy had an addiction: Facebook ads. Ads for supplements targeted to her demographic that fed into her belief of how she *should* be feeling, not into how she was actually feeling.

This is what the ads do. The algorithms are brilliant. All the ads that kept popping up on Suzy's feed told her and countless others like her to take 'X' supplement so she could feel better. That she absolutely needed 'X', or she was at risk of being unhealthy. She sent me links to the supplements on a regular basis, asking me what I thought. *"Should I be taking this?" "It says it's good for hair growth."* Or, *"It says my body doesn't make this, and I need it for more energy. What do you think?"* She was starting to get anxious, and it was making her feel bad about herself.

Note: The more anxious you become, the more havoc is wreaked on your gut.

Here's the thing. There will *always* be a product that claims to be the magic pill.

And everyone is jumping on the bandwagon.

That's why you have to get connected. Get connected to you, your body and what it is trying to say to you. It's about becoming familiar with the sensations that you are feeling and sensing, and what that means to you. We are so busy that we are in our heads. This exercise is an opportunity to create space for you. As you practice, you'll start developing a heightened awareness of the different sensations you are experiencing, and this is great information that will help you map out your inner guidance system.

PART II.
THE G.U.T. METHOD®

Get connected to your symptoms,
what you're thinking, how you're feeling.

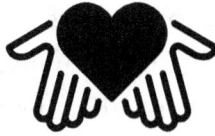

CHAPTER 5

MIND-BODY SCAN

••

"Your body is not a temple, it's an amusement park.
Enjoy the ride."

—*Anthony Bourdain*

••

Becoming aware and getting connected is the first step towards healing. There are a few components, and we're going to start with the physical body. The best way to start is by learning how to do a body scan on yourself. This helps you be present with you and your body. Pick a time of day that works for you to do this exercise (you'll start to notice a theme throughout the book about it working for you and fitting into your lifestyle). Maybe it's first thing in the morning, maybe it's before bed. Most of my clients like lying in bed so they can feel more relaxed but sitting in a chair with your hands resting on your lap, feet on the floor (not crossed) works as well. Pick a comfortable position. Find a place where you can have some quiet time; so, if you have young kids, you may want to wait until they go to sleep.

Sit (or lay) quietly with your eyes closed, breathing into your body and feeling it, and asking yourself questions. Remember, this exercise is to help you tap into *you*. You're not looking to define what it means. Not yet. We'll discuss that in a later chapter. Right now, you're simply working on getting connected, becoming aware, so that you can become more intuitive with understanding your body.

Read this next section first and then put the book down and follow the exercise. It should take about 5-10 minutes. Just notice what the time is when you start, and when you end. And don't worry as you do this exercise if you forget a section. This will be an ongoing practice that will help you relax, connect to and become aware of yourself, your body and your senses, and will become a tool for you to use when you feel overwhelmed, stressed out and anxious.

Close your eyes and start by breathing naturally in through your nose and out through your mouth. Feel your heart beating. Feel your muscles start to relax. Soften your mouth, letting your jaw relax. Let's start with awareness of your senses.

Let's start with *sound*: your ears. Notice the noise around you. Is it loud? Quiet? Sit with it and allow it flow through you as you continue to breathe. Do you hear any ringing or other sounds? Maybe air conditioning or the car horn outside, or even the birds chirping. Just notice the sounds around you.

How about your nose? Does it feel clear when you breathe in? Or is one or both nostrils clogged? Breathe through this a few times and observe. Maybe you have the sniffles, or your nose is running. Do you notice any smells? Perfume, cologne, air freshener. Just notice.

Let's move to *touch*: Feel the weight of your body on the chair, the clothes you are wearing. Just notice.

Move to your *mouth*: Does it feel dry? Do you taste anything? Maybe the tuna fish you ate for lunch (must have a little fun with this). Take a few breaths, noticing, becoming aware. How does your throat feel? Swallow a few times. Does it feel fine? Dry? Do you have a little cough? Maybe you're clearing your throat?

Now, let's move on to the rest of your body: *neck, chest, arms, hands, fingers, stomach, hips, legs, feet, toes.* Do you feel calm or restless? Are you relaxed? Tired? Do you feel any tingling anywhere in your body, your fingers, legs?

Keep breathing as you go through this. Just notice what you are feeling.

Where is your *mind*? If it feels like there are a dozen thoughts running through it, just notice it and bring the breath back to one of your five senses.

What are you feeling in your *stomach*? Gassy? Distended? Is it gurgling? If so, are you asking yourself if you're hungry? You'd be surprised with the conversations we start having with ourselves!

Scan every inch of your body.

WRITING EXERCISE
DIGEST AND DISCOVER

When you are done, think about what occurred and also
whether you feel more relaxed, or maybe even have a burst
of energy. Take some time to write your thoughts below.
Remember, this is about observation. Write this down
without judging what it means. For example: *My head feels
relaxed, a little heavy. I feel a little spasm in my neck. My
heart is beating slowly. I could hear the hum of the A/C, etc.*

_____

_____

_____

_____

_____

_____

_____

_____

_____

_____

_____

_____

_____

_____

_____

_____

_____

_____

_____

_____

_____

Now, record thoughts that came to you while you were developing answers. Our minds wander constantly. Maybe you started thinking about all the work you have to do, or the laundry or the e-mails you have to send. Be kind to yourself and just notice what your thoughts were.

_____

_____

_____

_____

_____

_____

_____

_____

_____

_____

Practice this exercise daily, noting where you may feel shifts in your body.

Symptoms

The next part of the body scan is about noticing any symptoms you are feeling that you may not be aware of or conditions that you may have. I've included a checklist below of physical symptoms for you to take some time and see what you may be experiencing now or in the last week. This is a judgment-free zone. Remember, it's about getting connected and just becoming aware. I don't want you to start thinking, *oh my God, I've checked off a dozen things here, and what does it mean?* We're *connecting* to our bodies and becoming *aware* of the different ways our bodies talk to us, and you'll see as you go through the next few chapters how you are going to put all the pieces together.

Abdominal pain		Dry mouth	
Acid reflux		Dry skin	
Acne		Ear infections	
Anal itching		Eczema	
Anemia		Excessive mucus in nose	
Anxiety / Anxiety attacks		Excessive mucus in throat	
Asthma		Excessive sweating	
Bleeding gums		Eye twitches	
Bloating after meals		Faintness/light-headedness	
Body odor		Fatigue	
Brain fog/trouble concentrating		Fearfulness	
Brittle/cracking nails		Foul smelling gas or stool	
Bruise easily		Gas	
Bumps on backs of upper arms		Hair loss	
Burping		Hair thinning	
Canker sores		Hay fever	
Clearing throat frequently		Headaches	
Cold sores		Heartburn/Indigestion	
Cold/Flu (frequent)		Hemorrhoids	
Constipation		Hives	
Cough – dry or phlegmy		Hot flashes/ Night sweats	
Cracked/splitting nails		Insomnia	
Cracks in corners of mouth		Irregular heartbeat	
Dandruff		Irregular periods	
Dark circles / bags under the eyes		Irritability / Easily agitated	
Depression		Itching	
Dermatitis		Itchy ears	
Diarrhea		Joint pain	
Difficulty concentrating		Joint stiffness	
Difficulty falling asleep		Joint swelling	
Difficulty gaining weight		Low libido	
Difficulty losing weight		Migraines	
Dizziness		Mood swings	

Muscle cramps / Stiffness		Rosacea	
Nausea/Vomiting		Salt cravings	
Nose bleeds		Sciatica	
Numbness or tingling		Sinus infections/problems	
OCD or obsessive thoughts		Sleepy during the day	
Oily skin		Snoring	
Panic attacks		Sore throat	
PMS		Spoon-shaped nails	
Poor concentration		Stuffy nose	
Poor memory		Sudden weight loss	
Premature grey hair		Sugar cravings	
Psoriasis		Sweating	
Rapid heartbeat		Tendonitis	
Rash		Trembling/shaky	
Redness of face, ears, nose		Waking up in the middle of the night	
Restless legs		Watery, itchy eyes	
Ridges on nails		White coating on tongue	
Ringing in ears		Yeast infections (athlete's foot, nail fungus, vaginal yeast infection, candida, etc.)	

Notes:

_____

_____

_____

_____

_____

_____

_____

_____

_____

_____

Next up: Your bowel movements. Yup! Your poop. I have to say, I never thought talking about poop would be part of my almost daily repertoire, but here we are.

Your stool has so many secrets and if you were to take an at home test through a functional nutritionist or doctor, you'd be surprised at the extensive information you would receive from the usual parasite, *H pylori*, to autoimmune triggers, inflammation and immune response. These tests are fascinating! But before you even know if you need that, you have to determine what your symptoms are and what your major health complaints are and speak to a professional if you have questions.

Below is a description of each stool type from the Bristol Stool Chart. Keep track of your bowel movements:

- **Type 1:**
  Separate hard lumps (very constipated)

- **Type 2:**
  Lumpy and sausage-like (slightly constipated)

- **Type 3:**
  Sausage shape with cracks in the surface (NORMAL)

- **Type 4:**
  Like a smooth, soft sausage or snake (NORMAL)

- **Type 5:**
  Soft blobs with clear-cut edges (lacking fiber)

- **Type 6:**
  Mushy consistency with ragged edges (inflammation)

- **Type 7:**
  Liquid consistency with no solid pieces (inflammation and diarrhea)

WRITING EXERCISE
DIGEST AND DISCOVER

Now, let's look at any emotional symptoms you are feeling. Write down what you are feeling and also, how often you may feel that way.

acceptance	capricious
admiration	caring
adoration	cautious
affection	certain
afraid	cheerful
aggravation	compassion
aggressive	complacent
agitation	compliant
agony	composed
agreeable	conceited
angry	concerned
anguish	confident
annoyance	contempt
anticipation	content
anxiety	crabby
apprehension	crazed
assertive	critical
assured	cross
awe	doubtful
bitter	dejected
bold	depressed
calculating	determined
calm	eager

easy-going	indecisive
ecstatic	inspired
elation	irritated
embarrassment	joy
emotional	longing
enjoyment	love
enraged	loving
enthusiasm	mad
envious	nervous
exasperation	optimistic
excited	peaceful
exhausted	pessimistic
extroverted	powerful
exuberant	resentful
fear	shame
fed up	shy
feeling like crying	stressed
focused	tired
frustrated	uncertain
grateful	weepy
hateful	worried

You probably weren't expecting that long list of emotions.

Still, I have good news. You are okay! The items you checked off are signs your body is talking to you and you'll see as we go through the second and third sections, that health status has many displays and this checklist is important to make sure that you take care of your biggest asset: you! These symptoms are there to let you know that something is going on internally, physically and emotionally. Chances are it is your gut (intuition) talking to you, telling you that it's time to pay attention.

We all want to have more energy and less stress. We all want to feel more joy. And we want deeper, more meaningful relationships and connection, whether it's with your significant other, parents, siblings, kids, friends or co-workers. Connection and community are integral to our growth: spiritually, emotionally, physically and mentally.

In order to get there, you have to start with building your own community within yourself with more self-compassion, less self-sabotage. More inner guidance, less listening to noise. More trusting your gut, less eating advertisements.

Write it down. Even if you think it's normal. I also encourage you to think about what conditions you may have been diagnosed with and write those down. This exercise isn't about judging or deciding. It's about observing your body. Getting in touch and getting connected. Did you notice any patterns? Did anything surprise you? Take some time to jot down your thoughts, and don't worry, you're not going for a Pulitzer here!

_____

_____

_____

_____

_____

_____

_____

_____

_____

Sometimes, exercises like this make people uncomfortable. I've gotten blank stares, nervous laughter, and a few mouth drops, as though I have two heads on my shoulders. We're not accustomed to taking this kind of time for ourselves.

Consider Evelyn. She's a type A lawyer who has been dieting for as long as she can remember. When we started working together and talking about taking time to complete this exercise, she laughed at me. We were talking via Zoom. I smiled and let the laughter settle down without saying a word. She stopped laughing and said, "You're serious, aren't you?" I nodded. Indeed, I was.

Then I noticed that she started to squirm in her chair. I invited her to share how this was making her feel. Her reply? *"Honestly? I think this is ridiculous. What is this going to prove?"* (Spoken like a true lawyer.)

One thing I love about working with my clients is that they know they have the space to be honest (as long as they're respectful). Her response was, respectfully, honest. I didn't take it personally. It's how she felt. Evelyn wasn't telling me that I was being ridiculous. She was just uncomfortable with the idea and attached an emotion to it. She could not fathom by any stretch of the imagination how this exercise could possibly help, but she was open to possibilities and trying.

SUCCESS   SUCCESS

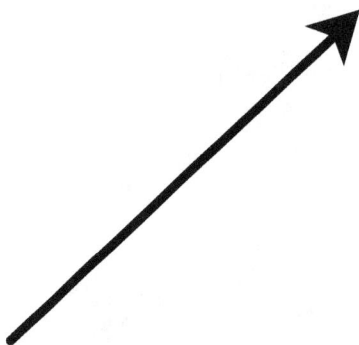

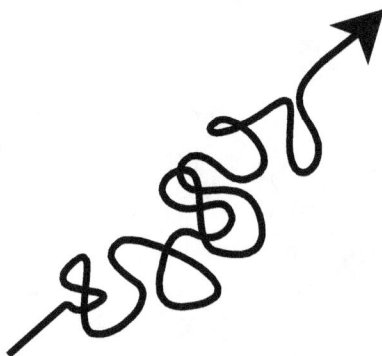

what people think   what it really
it looks like   looks like

What this scan does is put you in touch with yourself, right here, right now. It *connects* you to the present so that you can focus on your senses, your emotions and your body. You don't have time to think about the past or the future. You're here in the now. "Rome wasn't built in a day!" Your body (which includes your mental, physical and emotional state) didn't get to where it is overnight and feeling better, along with everything else, takes time. It's putting one foot in front of the other...one step at a time. You may take a couple of steps backwards, maybe even sideways along the way, but you will be going in a forward direction. It could look as messy as this diagram.

As Evelyn and I discussed the benefits of this exercise, she relaxed...a little. "Commit to it every day for one month, and then let's talk," I suggested.

She agreed, and you know what? Within a few weeks, she e-mailed me to let me know that she felt as though she was learning a new language and couldn't believe the questions it started to raise about how she had been living. The foods she chose, the relationships she had, her anger towards certain people as a result of expectations gone wrong, her type A personality at work. The assumptions she had made about certain situations in her life. The stress it was creating in her body and the choices she was making to nourish her body as a result. She started to realize that the conversations she was having with herself were so rooted in her wanting to protect herself, and her expectations of others, and she was judging herself (that's the ego, and we'll go into this in the *Understanding* chapter).

Evelyn had two reactions: she got scared and excited. So many thoughts were going through her head. *I want to do this but it's a little scary. You're challenging me go to places I have been suppressing for years and I'm all over the place, but I feel as though I really need to do this. On the other hand, I'm excited because I feel a shift happening—like there are so many possibilities that I wasn't aware of. I'm starting to look at situations and life with a different lens and realizing I've been playing the same tape in my head, but I've been running around in circles!*

Oh boy, could I relate to that and it can feel overwhelming. I recommended that she start writing down everything. It didn't have to be an essay. Bullet points, short sentences, anything to help her get all those thoughts and feelings out of her head and onto paper. She practiced writing without attaching judgment or blame, just with awareness.

That's all I ask of you right here and now. Practice this Mind/Body Scan as often as you can, working yourself up for a daily practice. Know that there may be days where you're in a groove and there may be days you have no desire to do it. It's okay! Remember, forward, sideways, backwards and forwards again. It's never a straight line and it will never be perfect. We're aiming for progress, not perfection.

I also recommend putting this on your calendar with an alert to help you remember. The more you practice, the easier it will get. Before you know it, you'll have a new habit. Before you know it, you'll see how you are creating your manual for your body and your life and you'll be able to refer back to it on occasions when life throws you a curve ball.

What Do You Taste Now?

In addition to getting connected to your symptoms and the way your body *feels*, I also want to introduce getting connected to your food at mealtime. We are a society that is always in a rush. To get to school. To drop kids off at daycare. To get to work. To catch a train. The list goes on. And with that, when it comes to eating, we don't "have time" to sit down and eat. We yell at our kids to hurry up because we're going to be late. We skip breakfast or grab a latte and a muffin, eat lunch at our desk and rush home to make dinner or order in. (Although at the time of this writing, we are in the midst of a pandemic that has actually given us our time back. Shelter in place to stay alive. Cooking and baking more than we may have ever done before. Dishwashers being used for the first time.)

All of the running around creates tension in our bodies and we end up gulping our food instead of chewing. Are we even tasting anything?

When I conduct workshops about this topic, I invite the audience to participate in an interactive experience using crackers (always offering a variety for those who are nut-free, gluten free or have other health concerns). Everyone takes two crackers. I tell them to eat one. That's it. Just eat your cracker. Then I ask for volunteers to share how many times they chewed the cracker. The answers range from "I don't know" to five to maybe 10. Then I ask what they tasted in the cracker. *Crickets*. Next, I ask them to eat the second cracker and chew at least 20-30 times. I ask again for volunteers to share what they tasted. More hands go up and people start sharing flavors that they tasted or that it got really mushy in their mouth and it was weird.

Connection and awareness to food. Slowing down gives you the opportunity to savor what you are eating. Do you even like what is on your plate?

At mealtime, it gives you and those you eat with time to, relax, have conversations and *connect to each other.* We all crave connection and if we can start with connecting to self, we can become more present, more aware, and that may open the door to so much more.

I want to encourage you as you read this book to take this action step right now while you get connected. It's as simple as making the choice to sit down for your meals, taking a few breaths to relax and chewing your food. With each meal, take a small bite (or fork-full or spoonful) and chew…aiming for 20-30 chews per bite.

Chewing is so important. It slows you down. It gives your brain and your gut time to communicate. The brain receives signals from the digestive hormones in the gut. Studies show that the slower you eat, the fewer calories you consume because your body will let you know that you are full, and this could lead to weight loss. In addition, the *British Medical Journal* shared research indicating that eating slower can inhibit the development of obesity. And it can start just with the act of chewing.

Digestion begins in the mouth and the more you chew, the smaller the particles become and the more surface area there is for enzymes to mix with saliva to start breaking down your food. I'll get more into this and understanding digestion in Chapter 9, but knowing that there is an action step you can take now, even if it's just one meal a day, you are taking steps to a healthier you as you think, eat and thrive.

THE G.U.T. METHOD®

Get connected to your symptoms,
what you're thinking, how you're feeling.

CHAPTER 6

FOOD JOURNAL

••

"Pull up a chair. Take a taste. Come join us.
Life is so endlessly delicious."

—*Ruth Reichl*

••

Keeping a food journal. Sounds so thrilling! Here's the part that has my clients roll their eyes at. You may be doing that as well. As I keep saying, this is a judgment-free zone! I didn't love keeping a food journal either. I hated it. Seriously. I didn't get it at first, so I used to think, *why bother, I'll remember everything, and I don't have time for this.* In reality, when I first started without writing, I couldn't even remember what I had for breakfast that day let alone the day before. But it's not just about what you are eating. It's also about getting a peek into your habits around food.

Our habits are unconscious and by looking at some of the foods we eat, the mindless snacking while we watch TV, we'll acquire insight and be able to shift our perspective to form healthier habits that serve us.

Once I started, I understood the value and also understood that over time, I wouldn't need the food journal once I connected to and became aware of my body. I realized I had to create new habits, and a food journal was the best and fastest way forward. Now that you are connecting to your body, its vital that you connect to the foods you eat and how they are (or aren't) serving you.

Let's start with what happens before you eat. Questions to start asking yourself are: Am I hungry, bored nervous, stressed, sad, anxious? Am I thirsty? Am I craving something salty? Sweet? Sour? Tangy? Fried? Am I eating because the clock says it's lunch time or my body says it's lunch time? Am I snacking a lot? Just observe.

When you eat, pay attention to what you are feeling in your body after one hour, three hours, even twenty-four hours. Are you: Bloated? Gassy? Constipated? Did your meal send you to the bathroom with diarrhea? Are you burping? Do you have heartburn?

Are you more tired?

Symptoms may not appear right away. Go back to the symptoms checklist. What is your gut saying? What are you *feeling*? What is that inner voice saying?

Write it all down. The beauty of these exercises is that you are creating your map with a key that will unlock the mysteries of your concerns, so that when we get to the section on understanding, you'll be able to refer back to your notes and start to notice patterns. Once you have the patterns and are able to connect the dots, then you'll be able to take action. You'll be able to tune in, trust yourself and take the appropriate steps to heal your body.

There are many ways to keep a food journal and you have to find the one that is right for you. Lately, most of my clients are finding it easier to just take pictures of their meals and snacks and drinks and putting them in to a word document and keeping notes that way. If you are visual, that's a great option. Some like to write it down on paper or laptop or mobile device. Some people are techies and like to use apps. Awesome! If you do choose to use an app, a few things to keep in mind: It is easy to get obsessed with the numbers. Many apps calculate the number of calories you need by asking for your height and weight and level of exercise. Once you see the number of calories it recommends for you, it may get embedded subconsciously, which may lead to obsession and confusion. Then the app asks you to fill out your food journal. It gets tricky if your item is not on their list or you may type in salmon and a dozen options pop up. This can get frustrating.

It also gets tricky when you have to fill out the exercise section because in some apps, if what you do is not on the list, you have to create it, and if you take classes like Barre or Pilates, you may have to build it in yourself. How the heck am I supposed to know how many calories the hundred in Pilates or the water-skiing exercise in Barre burns? Even if you choose to use the elliptical, it will ask you to input the number of calories burned, and if you're not wearing any type of monitor, but instead are relying on the machine, well, those numbers are rarely accurate.

I would also be mindful of how the macronutrients (fat, protein, carbohydrates) are broken down. For instance, when I played around with one app, in the nutrients section, it showed that I had eaten only 60 grams of my 110 grams goal of protein. But then, when I went to the macros section, it said that I had hit my goal of protein at 20%. Confusing? It sure as heck is to me and I'm a nutritionist! Stressful? I think my blood pressure just went up writing this! What do I listen to? Which one is more important? What do I do?

And the kicker for me...one app said that if I continued to eat this way (the way I had entered on that particular day), I'd weigh 11 pounds less in 5 weeks. Really? Well, I have news for that app. I eat like that pretty regularly and that scale did not budge one pound! The app has no idea what my stress levels are or my hormone levels, or if I need to lose weight, so how could it calculate that correctly? Right away, I'm thinking *this sucks.* I can only imagine what you may be thinking. "Calgon, take me away!" (If you're not familiar with that commercial, it ran back in the 70s, showing a person who has too much on her plate and has to escape and relax, and does so with a bubble bath.) This is why you have to do you. You have to figure out what is best for your body and your life (yup, I sound like a broken record).

I'd like to invite you to create a food journal that works for you. One that not only gives you space to enter the info, but also, space for comments on how you are feeling, stress levels, and other items. And as far as counting calories, don't. Period. I'll talk more about what your plate should look like in the *understanding* section.

I was at a networking event one evening and there was a panel of wellness experts talking about health and wellness in the corporate world. They had different businesses from meditation to dancing, to exercise and nutrition. What's interesting is the one thing they had in common: They talked about how disconnected we are from ourselves and those around us. How disconnected our minds and thoughts are from the rest of our bodies and how we need to tune in to ourselves and how important it is to our physical and mental health and our social wellbeing. *Yes!* Connection. We all want more of that, and here we are starting with *connecting* and becoming aware of your body.

To help you figure out what type of journaling works best for you, below is an example of one that I give to my clients. Take a look at it. Feel free to use it.

DAY ONE

Day Event	Food & Drink Intake (include type, amount, brand)	Describe how you felt after eating (tired, sluggish, etc.)
Rising Time		
Breakfast		
Mid–AM Snack		
Lunch		
Mid–PM Snack		
Dinner		
PM Snack		
Bed Time		

Sleep & Relaxation	Sleep	Relaxation
	Hours:	Yes / No
	Qualiy:	Type / Amount:

Exercise & Movement	Type, Duration & Intensity
	Aerobic:
	Strength:
	Flexibility:

Stress	Stress Reduction Practice	Stressors

Relationships	Supporting	Non-Supporting

Mental	
Emotional	
Spiritual	

In addition to this, below is a list of descriptions that describe your experience 1-2 hours after a meal (or in some instances, the next morning) that you can use in conjunction with the food journal.

Appetite	Feel full, satisfied
	Do NOT have sweet cravings
Satiety	Do NOT desire more food
	Do NOT feel hungrier
Cravings	Do NOT need to snack before next meal
Energy Levels	Renewed energy
	Good, lasting sense of energy
Mind	Clear thinking
Emotions	Feeling renewed, restored
	Emotional uplift, happy
Well Being	Improved mental clarity

Appetite	Feel physically full, but still hungry
	Have desire for something sweet
Satiety	Not satisfied
	Still hungry
Cravings	Feel like I need a snack
Energy Levels	Not enough energy
	Became hyper, jittery, nervous
	Feel exhausted, sleepy, lethargy
Mind	Slow, sluggish, spacy, brain fog
Emotions	Inability to think clearly or quickly
	Apathy, depression, withdrawal, sadness
Well Being	Anxious, obsessive, fearful, angry, irritable

WRITING EXERCISE
DIGEST AND DISCOVER

Use the space below to journal what you've discovered about yourself so far.

_____

_____

_____

_____

_____

_____

_____

_____

_____

_____

_____

_____

_____

_____

_____

_____

_____

_____

_____

_____

_____

_____

_____

Now that you've done your body scans, checked off some items on the checklist, started chewing your food, and have started keeping a food journal, I want to add more layers, which are equally as important to your health: your soul, your relationships and your mindset. We're setting up a complete foundation, getting connected and becoming aware of mind, body and spirit, and you'll see as you move through The G.U.T. Method®, how these pieces all fit together.

THE G.U.T. METHOD®

Get connected to your symptoms,
what you're thinking, how you're feeling.

CHAPTER 7

YOUR SOUL AND LOVE FOR SELF

∙∙

"The soul, fortunately, has an interpreter—often an
unconscious but still a faithful interpreter—in the eye."

—*Charlotte Brontë*

∙∙

When I was young, I couldn't wait for the Book Mobile
to come to our neighborhood. The Book Mobile was our
library on wheels, and I would wait impatiently every
Wednesday evening for this huge RV-style truck to come
rumbling down our street. I would race to it, wanting to
be the first one to board. It always felt like I was being
transported in time, whenever I climbed up those steps. As
I opened the door, the musty smell of books would come
wafting out and a big smile would cross my face. In my
mind, I was entering a time machine.

I was always drawn to mystery novels, the supernatural and at the time, Nancy Drew books or books on magic and witches. Maybe I really was a witch in a past life.

I share this with you because looking back, my soul felt nourished. Reading filled my cup. Escaping into these novels helped me cope with my life, although back then, I was too young to truly understand that it provided me with the escape I needed or that I was even looking for it because it was so unconscious.

Of course, when I got older, Nancy Drew books were replaced with wine. Red wine. Lots of it. My former husband and I owned a custom picture-framing store when our kids were little and right next to us was a liquor store. Every weekend, they had wine tastings. There was my bait. They had me hook, line and sinker. And once a month, a case would come home with me. It would take years for me to put the pieces together that I was self-medicating and it was affecting my nourishment—not only my physical health, but also, my soul's health.

Unconsciously Incompetent

Did you ever have a puzzle book where you connected the pieces to uncover what the picture on the page was supposed to be? Sometimes they were numbered; sometimes they were on a grid. To me, the pieces, or dots, are your symptoms. You get individual clues, but don't see the full picture until they are connected.

My body left me a trail of dots, symptoms that I wasn't paying attention to. They didn't mean anything to me because I didn't see the whole picture. They were just dots that I could sweep under the rug.

I remember one day turning on the TV, and Joel Osteen, an American pastor and author, was on. I had never heard of him, but something, a voice, told me to watch. I'm not Christian or religious, but there was something about Osteen's message that spoke to me. He talked about adversity and how sometimes we don't always know right away why we were dealt our hand, but if you pay attention, opportunities present themselves to elevate our souls. To some, this may sound like BS, but it felt as though he was talking right to me. Heck, he was even looking at me through my TV set.

He piqued my curiosity. I felt that there was an undulating wave, waiting for me to hop on the surfboard and ride it to a different shore to see what I would uncover.

I went to the bookstore and perused the self-help section in the hopes that something would stick out. My eyes scanned the titles as I ran my hand along the spines of the books. Something would say, "Read me!" I started with Wayne Dyer, Deepak Chopra, Louise Hay, and other spiritual thought leaders. I was finding a way back to my soul that was right for me. That was nourishing me. That was helping me put the oxygen mask on myself first so that I could be present, aware, in my life.

Your soul knows.

In essence, that means that so do you. That inner voice, that inner being that talks to you, is your soul. It's your inner emotional guidance system giving you information. It wants you to get connected and is trying to show you the way. You just have to be still enough to listen. When you do, and you hear the messages over and over, your gut, your inner knowing, will be able to guide you to make the right choices for you. All anyone can do, me included, is offer guidance. Some things will resonate more than others. That's the beauty of this journey and the more you allow yourself to open up and be vulnerable, the easier it will be to listen to those whispers, the easier it will be to feel love and joy from within. Follow the path of least resistance and allow your soul to sing.

Relationships Are Priceless—Continually Polish

Remember that WHO defines health as physical, mental, and social wellbeing, and as a resource for living a full life.

Relationships are part of that social and mental wellbeing. *All* relationships. With your parents, spouses, significant others, siblings, kids, friends, colleagues (even pets!) and yourself. This is an important part of getting connected because if we are to have meaningful relationships with others, we need to connect to and understand our relationship to ourselves and as we grow, it evolves and expands.

At first glance, this sounds abstract. If someone were to have asked me ten, fifteen, twenty years ago what my relationship with myself was, I'm sure the New Yorker in me would have flipped the person the finger, or at the very least, used a few expletives. *Relationship with self? What does that mean? And so what? Who cares? I'm fine with myself! Aren't I?* Unfortunately, in the world we live in today, we are so disconnected from ourselves. We might as well be walking around with our head in our hands because our mind and our bodies are not communicating.

As you've worked on getting connected to physical and emotional symptoms, you may have had a few epiphanies about yourself and your awareness may already be starting to shift.

Take a step away from that for a minute and let's go back to that contract you signed for yourself at the beginning of this book. Committing to honoring your body, to being open and believing in the possibilities of health, love and life. The path to getting where you want to go, begins with being honest with yourself; connecting to what you like and want or vice versa.

My client, the brilliant lawyer, keeps a self-talk journal. She wasn't so sure about it, but nonetheless, she decided to try it. In our work together, she became open to the possibility that there was much to learn about herself and this was the first step—writing down her thoughts, not analyzing them, just noticing them, becoming aware of them and the patterns, as well as how often she had the same thoughts and how they made her feel. She e-mailed me as I was writing this chapter to tell me that she now thinks in so many different ways, especially to see what is positive that is happening to her.

She added, "You generate such a good energy, and in my field, I really need that, so thank you."

I was so humbled by that statement. All I was doing was helping her, caring about her, and offering her the tools so that she can have a better relationship with herself as she continues on her journey to healing her body. This, in turn, has helped her heal hurt from a previous relationship. She was able to view the situation and circumstances objectively, without ego getting in the way and from that, she could release the pain and know that the person did the best they could, and she let it go.

The same client also told me that she had to buy exercise pants that were a size smaller. But the way she said it, she kind of threw it away, like tossing the baby out with the bath water. I made her stop and repeat her statement twice to emphasize how far she's come. "I suppose you're right. But I haven't reached my goal yet." It was the "but" that got me. It's an accomplishment. Pause and acknowledge it. Don't discard it as just another thing. It helps you generate more energy that starts to fill you and fuel you with excitement to keep going. That's why writing down the victories along the way, no matter how large or small, are so important. When your victories are on paper, you can see them, read them, and embed them in your soul. When the information is just in your head, you take the folder, file it somewhere in your brain, and forget about it because you are too busy putting out fires on a daily basis.

Also, it is so easy to be negative, to go down the dark alley and get swallowed up with thoughts that don't serve you. Warding them off requires consistency.

WRITING EXERCISE
DIGEST AND DISCOVER

Write down everything you can think of that has gone
right today, yesterday, last week, last month, even last year.
It could be as small as you drank more water today, to
something bigger, like having to buy a new pair of exercise
pants that are a size smaller. It could be that you are so
thankful for being healthy when you see people being
diagnosed with cancer or having died of the coronavirus.
Or maybe you scored a promotion or are simply smiling
because the sun is out.

_____

_____

_____

_____

_____

_____

_____

_____

_____

_____

_____

_____

_____

_____

_____

_____

_____

As you complete this exercise, I want you to consider being kind to yourself, which emits an aura. An energy that other people feel. It reminds me of the movie "Inside Out." Riley is an 11-year-old Midwestern girl, whose world turns upside-down when she and her parents move to San Francisco. Riley's emotions, led by Joy, try to guide her through this difficult, life-changing event. However, the stress of the move brings Sadness (the blue emotion) to the forefront. She drags everyone down, appears to be depressed. Know any people like that? Now, what about Joy? She's bubbly, always coming up with ideas and looks at life as a glass half full. She exudes energy and you want to be around her. People sense this and so do you.

Think about the people you know and meet. Some people can just rub you the wrong way. You don't know what it is exactly, but there's just something: energy.

We all have it. Our bodies are filled with electricity. Sometimes we attract the right people and other times, we repel them, and vice versa. And there are times when we are with someone whose being just makes us feel calm. We don't know why, but we want to be around that person. What you're feeling is their energy, and when you can be still, and allow yourself to feel it, allow yourself to feel the calm in your gut, your body relaxes, you feel less stress and without even knowing it, you then send out waves of similar energy to those around you, which will enhance your relationships.

Your Mindset, Beliefs, Expectations and Perceptions

Mindset. You hear this word a lot. Adjust your mindset. Change your mindset. It's all about your mindset. Fixed mindset. Growth mindset. Closed mindset. Open mindset. But what is it really? And what's the big deal?

The term was coined by Dr. Carol Dweck, a psychologist, who is a leading researcher in the field of motivation and mindset. Mindset is the established set of attitudes held by someone. It's about whether you believe that your thoughts and traits are fixed and can't be changed or whether you believe that they can be developed and strengthened, like muscles in your body. You wouldn't wake up one day and go to the gym and lift 50 or 100 pounds of weight without training and building your body up to being able to do that. You would start with light weights and work out consistently so that over time you get stronger and work your way up.

That's the same premise when it comes to your health, your relationships, and your life. We sometimes get caught up in the outcome, in the future, instead of being present and focusing on what can be done today and then keeping track. The challenge that so many people have is that if there is too much going on in our heads, we'll forget the baby steps that we've taken that have gotten us this far. That leads us to focusing on what hasn't gone our way, instead of what has worked so far.

Every day, you get a chance to reset and move forward. But don't let that deter you if you feel like it's "Groundhog Day." Have you seen that movie? Bill Murray, a self-centered, superficial weatherman, who has a limited mindset, wakes up to the same day, every day. What they don't tell you in the movie is that he is stuck in the town of Punxsutawney for eight to ten years! This movie actually illustrates the concepts of Buddhism, and while I'm not here to proffer any religious views, there are a few universal truths you can take away from this movie: Be kind to others. Have an open mind. Try different things. In order to find love, you have to work on yourself. Life is what you make it.

At first, Bill's character, Phil, is annoyed, but in time, he realizes that it is an opportunity for him to shift his actions for a better outcome. Eventually, he gets to the finish line because he learns from his journey. Andy McDowell's character, Rita, at one point, says how she is completely amazed, and Phil asks about what. And she says how you can start the day with one expectation and end it completely different.

Expectations also exist around food, dieting, your relationships with friends, family and loved ones, but if you can focus on your perspective and figure out why you have a certain expectation, you'll have that power to make the shift, starting the day thinking one way and being pleasantly surprised with a different outcome. You have the power to change it. To get connected. To become aware. It just takes practice. It may have taken Phil ten years and it may take you ten years (or ten days or ten months), but you'll never know if you don't start.

This is your journey. There will be good days, great days and maybe not such great days, and if you write down what has worked so far, if you focus on all the good things that have happened, it gets easier to stay focused on your why, so keep that in mind.

Throughout this section of connection, it's important to have self-compassion. Self-compassion is the ability to show empathy; the ability to not only show love and concern to others, but also, to be able to direct those same emotions within and accept oneself, especially in instances of perceived inadequacy, failure, or general suffering. You may want to begin by reviewing your own life and asking yourself questions:

- What kind of person have I been?

- What do I say to myself if something doesn't go my way?

- Am I hard on myself?

- Do I use words that are negative or positive? Examples of this when it comes to food is the concept of the word 'diet' which can be defined as restricting the amount of food to lose weight.

- Who said you had to lose weight?

- Why do you have to weigh a certain amount?

- What happens when you 'cheat?' Do you beat yourself up? What if you stopped dieting? What would that feel like? What if instead of cheat, you use the word 'indulge?' Doesn't that sound better? Cheating makes me feel crappy, like I failed. But indulging provides room to allow without the guilt or shaming that we do to ourselves.

WRITING EXERCISE
DIGEST AND DISCOVER

Can you think of times when you were so critical of yourself yet so kind to others? Take time now to reflect on the words and phrases you think and use. Write them in the space below. If they are negative, let's reframe them to positive. (i.e. Negative: I have to diet the rest of my life or I'll gain weight. Positive: Diets don't work. I am going to re-evaluate what I need for my body so that I can stop dieting.)

_____

_____

_____

_____

_____

_____

_____

_____

_____

CHAPTER 8

FEEL AND HEAL!

....

"If you are always trying to be normal, you will never
know how amazing you can be."

—*Maya Angelou*

....

You are made up of trillions of cells: 50 trillion, in fact, asserts Dr. Bruce Lipton, in his book, *The Wisdom of Your Cells.* These cells are alive, which when you think about it, makes you a community, not just a single person. Every cell is electrically charged, like a battery and the human body produces energy equivalent to a 100-watt light bulb. Imagine then, that you can use that energy to heal.

In addition to that ability, all animals and all plants communicate through vibration. If we were taught when we were young to listen and to *feel* the vibrations and energy, we would have a deeper understanding of who we are as individuals and how to connect to our inner wisdom.

We would have a different outlook on health, relationships and life.

However, instead of being taught to listen to our feelings and to know, truly know, that we have the energy and vibration to *feel and heal* from within, instead of being taught to trust ourselves, we were taught to listen to and do what other people have to say and tell us. Instead of being taught to trust ourselves, we were taught to ask others what they think and then to trust their answers, and in doing so, we have become more disconnected from ourselves and others.

I'll never forget, when my oldest son, Evan, was around 2 years old, my former husband and I decided to hire a babysitter for Saturday nights, so that we could go out for the evening. During the interview process, I'd see how the person interacted with my son. One woman, who was an elementary school teacher, seemed sweet. Evan was unusually quiet, and while I noticed it, I didn't think much of it. Everything looked good on paper, she seemed nice, and she had been recommended by an acquaintance. We hired her.

The first Saturday evening, Evan hid behind my legs. Normal for a toddler. He asked us not to leave and we did the good-parent thing—reassured him that everything was okay, kissed him, and said goodnight. He cried as we left, and, while my heart sank, I kept telling myself that everything was fine. He was just being a toddler.

When we came home, Evan was asleep. We paid the babysitter and said goodnight.

The next morning, we asked Evan how he liked her. He shrugged his shoulders. I tried to ask him questions, but he was two years old! Wasn't going to get much out of that department! I shrugged it off, thinking, *he's a toddler.*

The following weekend came, and Evan started getting agitated. He cried for us to stay home when we told him the babysitter was coming. The doorbell rang and as soon as I opened the door, he clung to me and wouldn't let go. I could have peeled him off of me and reassured him that everything was okay, and that Mommy and Daddy were just going out for a few hours and we'd be home later, but I felt that something was off. *My knowing, my intuition, my gut, said, something isn't right here.* I asked her point blank, "Did you do something to Evan last week? He has never reacted this way to anyone."

I know I was accusing her and there was probably a better way to handle that, but Mama Bear was out in full force and no one was passing go. She looked annoyed and said she was a teacher; how could I even ask her that question.

That didn't deter me. Evan wouldn't let go. I could *feel* his fear and I felt that she was holding back information. Let's call a spade a spade. I was sure she was lying, but all I had was my son's reaction. His fear was proof enough. I looked at my former husband and said we couldn't leave Evan.

I paid her for four hours, told her we would not be using her as a babysitter again and closed the door. I then turned to my son and scooped him up. He trembled in my arms as I promised him she would never come to the house again. My heart sank. What happened? Did she hurt my son? While I would never know the answer, deep down, I know my intuition and understanding of that moment led me to making the right call for my son.

I realized there were subtle signs during the interview process and that first evening she babysat for us. My son had showed me his signs. He couldn't articulate it verbally, but he showed me physically. I didn't pick up on it at first, but fortunately, it didn't require another evening for me to understand and act.

In the movie, "Avatar," they say, "I see you," meaning, I see the love and your feelings and your soul. When you start to get connected, you're plugging into an existing energy source and a new level of vibration that allows you to truly see another without judgment or any type of emotion except love for the soul. They're vibrational waves that permeate the air. That's why one person can feel another person's energy, and know if something is off, when they're connected and tuned in. At first, I didn't see my son during those two episodes with the babysitter. I just wanted to go out. After that last episode, I saw him clearly, tuned in to his frequency and responded.

My awareness and understanding had been awakened. I needed to remind myself to pay more attention. It would take me another decade to get connected to my soul and my kids through Zach's diagnosis and my divorce.

Start Grasping, Stop Gasping

Your inner being, your intuition, gut instinct, whatever you want to call it, and the law of attraction have the capacity to bring you what you need. Now that you've started to get connected to different aspects of your health and your life, and as you become aware of what that looks like, let's understand how this is all connected.

Miriam Webster defines "understanding" as mental grasp...comprehension, a friendly or harmonious relationship; tolerant, *knowing.* It is sympathetically being aware of other people's feelings and your own.

There's so much to consider with understanding. Before I get to that *knowing* though, I want to walk you through a *simple* understanding of food, of macronutrients (protein, fats and carbohydrates), micronutrients (vitamins and minerals), how to look at your plate, and what to look for in nutrition labels. I find that this has become so obscured with all the different buzz words we hear such as *Keto diet, vegan, Paleo, low-carb, juicing, high in antioxidants, all natural, gluten-free, made with real fruit, no added sugar...*the list goes on and on. As I've mentioned in earlier chapters, when we hear messages over and over, we really do start to believe what the 'experts' are saying and what the ads are telling us.

Let's consciously arrive at a simple understanding of what we think we know, something we can always come back to for clarity.

There are six classes of nutrients: water, carbohydrates, fat, protein, vitamins and minerals. Your body is composed of approximately 60-75% water, according to researchers in the *Biological and Biomedical Sciences Program at Harvard Medical School,* and it is essential to life. You may have heard that you can survive a month without food but couldn't survive three days without water. It helps regulate body temperature, carry nutrients to our cells, flush out toxins and waste and so much more. It also influences the shape of cells, which is important for proper function. For instance, without the proper shape of protein, your body wouldn't be able to drive contraction of muscles, communication, digestion of nutrients and other vital functions.

Proteins are the primary material of life and are made up of amino acids. Proteins play an essential role in our bodies, ranging from regulation of gene expression and building muscle, to helping your hair and nails grow.

Carbohydrates provide your body with the energy it needs but all carbohydrates are not created equal. There are complex carbs (starch and fiber; very important to our *diet* - and simple carbs, or sugars). Sugar is a gargantuan topic, with many resources on it available, but since it affects our gut microbiome, I will address it for that reason alone. Evidence supports the notion that sugar, among other poor dietary factors, changes the gut microbiota in a way that increases intestinal permeability (i.e. leaky gut, which will be discussed in the upcoming chapters).

When we ingest sugar and refined carbohydrates, our blood glucose spikes and alerts our pancreas to produce the hormone, *insulin*. Insulin then tells our cells that it's time to "get energy" from the ingested sugar. Regular sugar intake can interfere with your endocrine function. Over time, this constant intake of added sugar and the roller coaster track can build insulin resistance. Insulin resistance is when the body and liver begin to store sugar as fat. Associations between increased risk of diabetes, heart disease, obesity, cancer, high blood pressure, cognitive disorders (e.g. dementia, Alzheimer's, etc.) and other conditions entailing impaired immune function and added sugar intake have been established.

Fats help your body absorb nutrients and certain vitamins as well as help your body produce hormones, bile and Vitamin D, as needed. You've heard about good fats and bad fats (and I almost feel like this should be a scene in the "Wizard of Oz" between the good witch and the bad witch), and they have been villainized over the years, which has confused us even more.

The Dietary Reference Intake (DRI) is 20%-35% of total calories coming from *healthy* fat. Do not remove this food group. I remember when I believed that low fat dieting was the way to go and figured if I had fat-free cookies, I was fine because there wasn't fat. (Yeah...I know!)

Vitamins and minerals are nutrients that the body needs to work properly. They help perform hundreds of roles, from bone growth, to protecting the body from birth defects and your vision, to immunity and more. This area gets tricky because we hear about supplements and may end up taking too many or the wrong ones for our bodies. Supplements are meant to be just that; supplement your daily intake of nutrients. Before hitting 'buy now', take stock on what you really need. You'll be able to figure this out through a combination of avenues starting with your symptoms checklist and looking to food first. If you experience symptoms that require the assistance of nutritional and medical help, then you'll expand to getting to the root with blood work, gut function testing, hair analysis, hormone testing, and maybe even as far as heavy metal and mold testing. It depends on your individual needs (and if you have acute symptoms or other medical need, don't hesitate and get help). *This is why connecting to and understanding your body is essential.*

Understanding what a plate should look like and how much of what foods to eat (oh my!) is always a question I get asked. As I've mentioned, we've been conditioned to count calories, eat less and exercise more. But it's not the calories we have to concern ourselves with. It's the nutrients. What is in those calories. An apple may have more calories than a bag of low-calorie chips but you're better off with the nutrient dense earth grown apple (organic when possible) than a bag manufactured in a facility that has been sitting on a shelf for months. Half your plate should be the colors of the rainbow in vegetables, ¼ for protein and the rest filled with slow burning carbs (i.e. root vegetables, brown rice) and healthy fats such as olive oil, nuts and seeds, avocado. I know that sounds general, but it's a good place to start.

What does your plate look like?

To give people an idea of labels and ingredients, I love to play another game at my speaking engagements. The game is Guess What. I put ingredients on the screen and ask the audience to guess what the food is that it makes. I always start with something simple like lettuce, cucumber, carrots, tomatoes. And everyone knows the answer: Salad.

Then I share a list of ingredients that is a mile long and everyone stares. No one can guess. Well, that's not true. There was one time when I spoke at a company and was pleasantly surprised that someone called out the correct answer. But most people gasp when they see what it is (you'll have to attend one of my workshops to see).

Awareness and understanding. If you can't understand most of the ingredients, then how does your body know what to do with that packaged food you're chewing.

That leads me to nutrition labels. I've shared throughout the first section how we've been conditioned to eat advertisements, on TV, the Internet and the marketing claims on products we buy at the supermarket. You may have heard that you should eat products with the fewest ingredients and be able to understand them. That's not enough. For example, there are brands of bars that are in the protein bar section that tout "fewer than 6 ingredients", and have the right buzz words, such as gluten-free, dairy-free, vegan, non-GMO, etc. The first thing to be aware of is the subliminal message that if we saw it in the protein bar aisle, it must indeed have enough protein and be good for us. And we may just grab it because we like the packaging or the buzz words. And it may indeed be all natural, even the sugars. But when you look at the nutrition label, there's more sugar than protein, fiber and fat! Just because something is natural doesn't mean it's truly healthy. What's important is if this bar is going to spike your blood sugar.

My client, Natalie, always took care of herself and was surprised to learn that she was pre-diabetic. While she ate a healthy diet, she loved protein bars and bananas. She wasn't getting enough fiber or essential fatty acids. She didn't understand that just those two foods could wreak havoc on her body. Once she was educated, she made small tweaks in her diet and everything changed. Once she swapped out the bananas for berries (she still ate a banana once in a while), stopped eating the bars and added more dark green, leafy vegetables, chia seeds and other high fiber foods, and even learned how to make her own protein bars (not as difficult as it sounds), her blood sugar stabilized. She was thrilled. And she had more energy. She thought she was just getting older and that was why she was tired every afternoon.

Now, that's a simple case and they're not all that easy, but it's always the place to start. Education and understanding what your body needs.

Another common food that gets overlooked are nut butters. Do you know why you buy what you buy? Is it price? Buzzwords? The story about the founders (who doesn't want to support the family-owned business!)? Next time you go the supermarket, look at the ingredients of some of your favorite brands. Nut butter should just have nuts and maybe sea salt. If yours has added sugar and oils, even if it says all natural, you have to ask yourself *why,* and do you really need it (and the answer here would be a resounding no). A little caveat: I'm not the food police. And I don't live in the woods and eat bamboo shoots and leaves and I don't expect you to either. The goal isn't to become obsessed with all the details, but to give you an understanding so that you can be educated to make the right decisions. And it doesn't mean that you have to be perfect.

You may have heard of the 80/20 or 90/10 rule. If you look at your week and plan your meals in a way that serves you, then if you eat nutrient dense foods 80%-90% of the time, there's always room to play. Maybe you want that protein bar, which is more of a glorified candy bar, or maybe you want to enjoy a cocktail or dessert when you're out to dinner. By giving yourself room to live, to enjoy life, you can have your cake and eat it, too. (Judge the size and maybe get a few forks and share it.)

Part of life is savoring our dinners and conversations with friends and loved ones. The more you can practice joy and occasional indulgence, without judgement, the more relaxed you will be and the easier the habits will be for you to create and incorporate into a lifestyle that works for you. Before you know it, you will actually start eating more intuitively, because you are finally connecting to your body and its needs!

Let's discuss one last item before heading back to that *knowing* that I mentioned at the beginning of this chapter: meals and mealtime. I'm frequently asked what to eat for breakfast. It's that one meal that everyone gets bored of quickly. We've been conditioned to think that breakfast comes in a box...of cereal.

A few facts about that box:

- Cereal was invented in 1863.

- There are over 100 different cereals on the market which account for $11 billion share of the food market.

- Each year, the cereal industry uses approximately 816 million pounds of sugar.

- Some US cereals are banned in other countries because of the use of certain dyes that are considered carcinogenic.

For those who have upgraded and moved away from cereal, the question then is what do I eat? For many who are moving away from dairy and refined grains, that could feel limited to oatmeal, non-dairy yogurt, shakes, and eggs.

What is breakfast and why do we get frustrated with what to eat?

Breakfast is Really Break Fast

You are breaking your fast from the night. Your body has had time to rest and digest. Other than that, breakfast is just a meal, like lunch and dinner. So, why limit yourself to the options mentioned above? Why continue buying into the notion that something in a box that has been sitting on a shelf for months is good for your body?

Here's the thing. You can make your own rules when it comes to food and what to eat. If you follow a sensible eating plan with healthy proteins, fats, fiber and a rainbow of vegetables and fruits, and staying properly hydrated, you're well on your way to nourishing your body and giving it the energy that it needs to sustain you and get your day started. The time that you eat depends on you, your body and your day.

I've had clients tell me they're not a breakfast person. Honestly, I'm not always a breakfast person either. It depends on many factors that each one of us has to learn about ourselves. You're okay! Maybe you ate early one day and at 5:00 p.m. you became ravenous. Instead of thinking *oh it's too early to eat dinner, let me have a snack*, why not just eat dinner at 5:00? Worried that you'll think you're turning into your grandmother who had to stand in line at the local deli for the five o'clock special? Who said dinner had to be at the time you were raised to believe? What matters is what you need (and what your family needs if you have one that you are living with).

Comprehension for Wellbeing

In order to understand, we have to break down what that word "understanding" means to us, how it appears within each of us. One aspect of understanding that has become so clear to me is how we each show up in any type of relationship, especially for those in a romantic one, because we each have our own baggage. We each learned how to love differently, whether it is through respect and admiration, showing affection and kindness, quality time together, touch, intimacy, words of affirmation, or to the other extreme of being manipulative or using guilt (check out the five love languages).

We need to understand the words we choose to communicate and whether those words are bringing us closer to our truth or further away from it. Whether we are feeling connected or disconnected. Whether we are being the light and energy for others or the fear and darkness. Whether we are lifting people up or bringing them down, and vice versa. Whether it is our ego or our authentic self.

How you view things is what will also help you to understand what the signs and symptoms that you worked on in the first section mean to you. What's important to this process is being open to receiving and allowing for a new understanding to pass through the gates.

Belief Systems

Did you believe in the tooth fairy when you were little? When your first tooth fell out, did you parents tell you to put it under the pillow and the tooth fairy would come, take your tooth and leave you some money?

When my twins were little, they asked questions about the tooth fairy, so my former husband suggested they write a letter to the tooth fairy and put it under their pillow with the tooth. He then got creative. He found a picture of a castle and put that on paper and typed up a letter back to whoever lost their tooth. The exchange between my kids and the tooth fairy took on a life of its own, as they became pen pals. While the idea was cute (they were so thrilled that the tooth fairy wrote to them and left them money with a letter!), I knew we were headed for disaster.

What I didn't expect was that I would be the one to burst the bubble. You see, one morning I had to leave early and Zach came running to me, saying that there was nothing under his pillow! I was in such a rush that I told him dad would give him money.

"What? Why would Dad give me money? What about the tooth fairy?"

O-M-G. What had I just done?

Why did I say that? All these thoughts quickly ran through my head. *I'm a terrible mother. It's not my fault. My former husband should not have started this. It's his fault. Will my kids hate me? Will they be forever be traumatized by their mother and the now, non-existent tooth fairy?*

I didn't have time, so I apologized to Zach, told him to go to Dad, and left the house feeling devastated that I had ruined their lives, and feeling bad (a little) knowing that my former husband would be left to clean up the mess (initially I thought, *well, it serves him right, he should never have started this,* but that was my ego speaking)!

We had trained our kids to believe in the tooth fairy. Simple. Innocuous. Fun. Traumatizing.

Beliefs. They're generally formed by our experiences or by accepting what others tell us to be true. While we are born without any preconceived notions of what beliefs are, most of our core beliefs are formed during our childhood years and what we experience and understand as we get older, helps shape who we are and what we become and that includes our expectations of others. Once we become aware of these beliefs and are open to receiving the new information, then we can create change in our lives.

Our psychological make-up is as different and individual as our fingerprints. Scientists who study epigenetics would even say it's been passed down through our DNA. The way we each handle situations is so unique, just as our guts and nutritional needs are, that we really need to understand ourselves individually, before we decide what course of action to take in all aspects of our lives.

There is no right or wrong answer. There is just 'what is' and what is right for you. If you want to live a keto or vegan *lifestyle*, it is not for me or anyone to judge you. Notice how I stress the word lifestyle. This is different than saying, "I'm going to *try* another diet."

WRITING EXERCISE
DIGEST AND DISCOVER

Understand what it is that you want and why. It has to work for you because you know your body best. Your why is so important. Why do you want to lose weight? What will that look like? How will that feel? Why do you feel like you have to count calories or diet all the time? Are you doing it for the right reasons or because it's what you've been trained to believe? Write down your thoughts.

_____

_____

_____

_____

_____

_____

_____

_____

_____

_____

_____

_____

_____

_____

_____

_____

_____

_____

_____

For me, my belief systems led me to understand that the "experts" knew everything and that I should listen to authority. I understood and believed what they said. Why wouldn't I? Weren't they trained to help? Be of service? Why would I think that they're deceiving me?

As I grew up, despite suffering from constipation most of my childhood, and IBS, and sinus infections and strep throat, and eczema, and sties, and migraines, and anemia, and heavy periods, (oh my!), I understood that if the doctors could give me medicine and they weren't alarmed, then it was all right and that I was all right and healthy.

I understood from magazines and the mean girls at school that "thin" was "in." And if I wasn't thin, then I had to diet and keep dieting, from the grapefruit diet in middle school to Dexatrim pills in high school. It became my "what is" and after a while I was on autopilot, detached and going through the motions to be thin. To weigh a certain amount on the scale. To have pants that were big. No matter whether I would hit my goal, I never felt thin enough or pretty enough and let's face it, I was never going to be in.

My understanding at that time was skewed with the information I had learned. It had become so ingrained in me that it became a fact, which was then my truth. I had given away my power and allowed what others thought and said become more important than what I thought and wanted. My perspective needed to shift in order for me to get connected, become aware that my old definition of understanding needed to change.

Perhaps yours does, also.

One of my clients, Pam, came to me originally because she wanted to lose weight, always felt bloated, was constipated, tired, stressed out, had headaches, insomnia, mood swings, hot flashes and daily cravings. She felt like she was losing control. I assured her that she was not alone and that many of my clients feel the same way. Married with kids and a demanding career, Pam was physically and emotionally barely scraping by. She had tried diets and diet pills, and nothing worked.

After filling out her intake form and going over her symptoms with her during our consultation, I recommended a couple of tests that she could do at home that would show us what was going on in her gut as well as what was happening with her hormones and cortisol levels. When we received the results, she was able to see how the results correlated with her symptoms. We discussed different options and after agreeing on the best course of action for her, she chose a protocol that she could implement given her busy lifestyle. This included food shifts, supplements, mindset, exercise, ways to improve sleep, stress-reducing strategies, and inner soul work.

During that time, we also discussed what was happening to her body and more importantly, *why*. No one had ever explained to her the why. She had been left to her own devices to Google everything and learn nothing because the information was so overwhelming.

As she started to get connected, the *understanding* of what she needed, what her body and her mind needed to heal became more apparent. In the first month alone, after swapping a few food options and adding a few supplements, she was amazed at how she went from being constipated to having bowel movements daily! The bloating was gone, and the headaches were decreasing. The following couple of months, she had more energy than she could remember. She gave up one of her biggest vices, coffee. She was sleeping better, cravings disappeared, and she felt like a different person.

Breaking news! Up until that point, she only lost four pounds and it didn't matter as much to her. She was so thrilled that she had so much energy, felt lighter, had no headaches, and that she was feeling so much more connected, to her body and herself, that her relationship with her spouse and her kids improved. She was more patient, she felt more at peace, and she knew the weight loss would come and that she probably didn't need to lose as much weight as she thought she did. Because she wasn't bloated and constipated anymore, her clothes fit so much better. She *felt more joy.*

Her understanding of why she was feeling the way she was feeling and finally being able to do what was right for her body that fit her lifestyle had created more space for her mentally and emotionally. Instead of worrying about her health, she was able to shift her focus and perspective on life, career and health to what was important for her and her family.

Another client, Chris, only 23 years old at the time that we started working together, was still in college and had severe IBS, a common disorder affecting the large intestine whose symptoms include cramping, bloating, gas, constipation or diarrhea or both, so much so that she had trouble going to class because she was always running to the bathroom. It kept her from being able to focus because she was always worried about her stomach acting up and not being near a bathroom. She was afraid of eating because everything seemed to set her bowels off. This didn't make for fun evenings out with friends. She had a colonoscopy and endoscopy (thankfully nothing showed up) and came to me through her mother, who was at her wit's end trying to help her daughter.

I get it. I not only went through it myself for years when I was younger; I had also experienced that with my son.

You know the saying, "You're as happy as your least happy child." When your child isn't feeling well, all you want to do is make it better and you can sometimes feel helpless when you've exhausted all options, and nothing works.

Chris conducted a stool test at home and when we sat down to go over her symptoms and the results, she understood through my explanation, what was going on in her body. She realized that in order to heal, she had to decide what she wanted and why. Was it worth staying in pain or worth putting the oxygen mask on herself so that she could heal and have more energy and feel better? She had a choice and she chose herself. She chose to feel well, and she began implementing the changes and upgrade her food choices. She healed within months and felt like a new person. Eighteen months later, she feels great! I checked in with her just today and she said, "I'm totally different from even this time last year. It's awesome!"

When you understand why, your whole perspective changes. You start having epiphanies and the clarity and understanding creates room for you to feel better, lighter, empowered and full of possibilities.

WRITING EXERCISE
DIGEST AND DISCOVER

Think about what you think you understand about your body, your symptoms and all the different modalities you may have tried in the past. What do you believe when it comes to ads and marketing claims? If you're dieting, what do you understand dieting to be? Why are you on a diet? What do you want your future self to look like and feel?

_____

_____

_____

_____

_____

_____

_____

_____

_____

_____

_____

_____

_____

_____

_____

_____

_____

_____

Understand that behind every feeling is emotion and emotion is the energy that moves you.

Understand that your body wants to be in alignment. It wants to feel balanced. It wants to feel great, and it's screaming at you to take care of it with compassion because you are the only one who knows you best.

Understand that your habits are 40-50% (conservatively) unconscious and with that, you may have unconscious expectations of yourself and others and that perhaps now is the time to explore why you became disappointed when things didn't work out the way you planned. You have the power to shift to the conscious level and start to change those thoughts and habits.

Understand that the universe is sending you the signs; that your body is sending you the signs, and that when you feel peace and balance, it feels calm. On the other hand, when you start to feel anxious and unsettled and hit resistance, this may be a sign that what you are doing or even the thoughts you are thinking are not in alignment.

The understanding is also allowing yourself to be vulnerable and brave at the same time. I learned this from Brené Brown, one of my favorite authors and speakers. To realize that it is your time now to get to the root.

Not too long ago, my oldest son was sharing a conversation he had with a friend (they are both in their late twenties). His friend was experiencing aches and pains and said to him, "I don't know if this is a thing, an injury, or if I'm just getting older."

At first, to my son, the idea that this friend may "just be getting older" sounded normal because of what we see and hear on TV and in magazines, we're conditioned to believe just that. But think about it. A young woman in her late twenties who thinks that she is in pain just because she is getting older is already setting herself up for failure because no one has told her that she shouldn't be thinking that way. I do not remember ever having a conversation in my twenties with anyone that remotely sounded like that. We were just getting started! We didn't feel like we were just getting older or that our bodies were falling apart (although, looking back, mine was).

Yet now, this is common. We are inundated with thousands of messages daily. Our minds have to sift through *a lot* of information and decide what to keep as important, what to store and what to discard. It creates a lot of anxiety, and the last thing it leaves us with is calm or peace or balance.

So, with all of this information, what can you do? How do we stop the madness? I want to start by first understanding what happens when we eat, how your body digests food, understand what leaky gut is, understand your gut microbiome, and why it's called your second brain, understand how it's not just food, but also stress, and toxins in products: those you put on your skin to products used to clean your house.

Before you get all nuclear on me, let me assure you that what you are going to read next is not what you'll find in biology class or in a chemistry lab. No degree is necessary. However, I think it is vitally important to have a simple understanding of all the components that are creating this chaos in your body. I've learned from my clients, and what they really appreciate most, is when we have our results and review session over Zoom or in person, that they enjoy learning about digestion, leaky gut and the microbiome, because that, coupled with their symptoms and the test results, really helps them visualize and understand what is happening in their bodies.

THE G.U.T. METHOD®

Get connected to your symptoms,
what you're thinking, how you're feeling.

CHAPTER 9

WHERE DOES IT ALL GO? AN *INSIDES* PRIMER

....

"He who conquers himself is the mightiest warrior."

—*Confucius*

....

Digestion

Ever notice how you begin to salivate when you smell something being baked in the oven? Interestingly, before you even take your first bite, your body is already getting ready to digest food just by the smell. Digestion starts in the mouth, where amylase enzymes (in your saliva), start to break down carbohydrates.

After chewing, the muscles in the wall of the esophagus help to propel the food to the stomach. In the stomach, a mixture of digestive enzymes and stomach acid, continue the work of digestion, and when the food is broken down sufficiently, it moves to the small intestine.

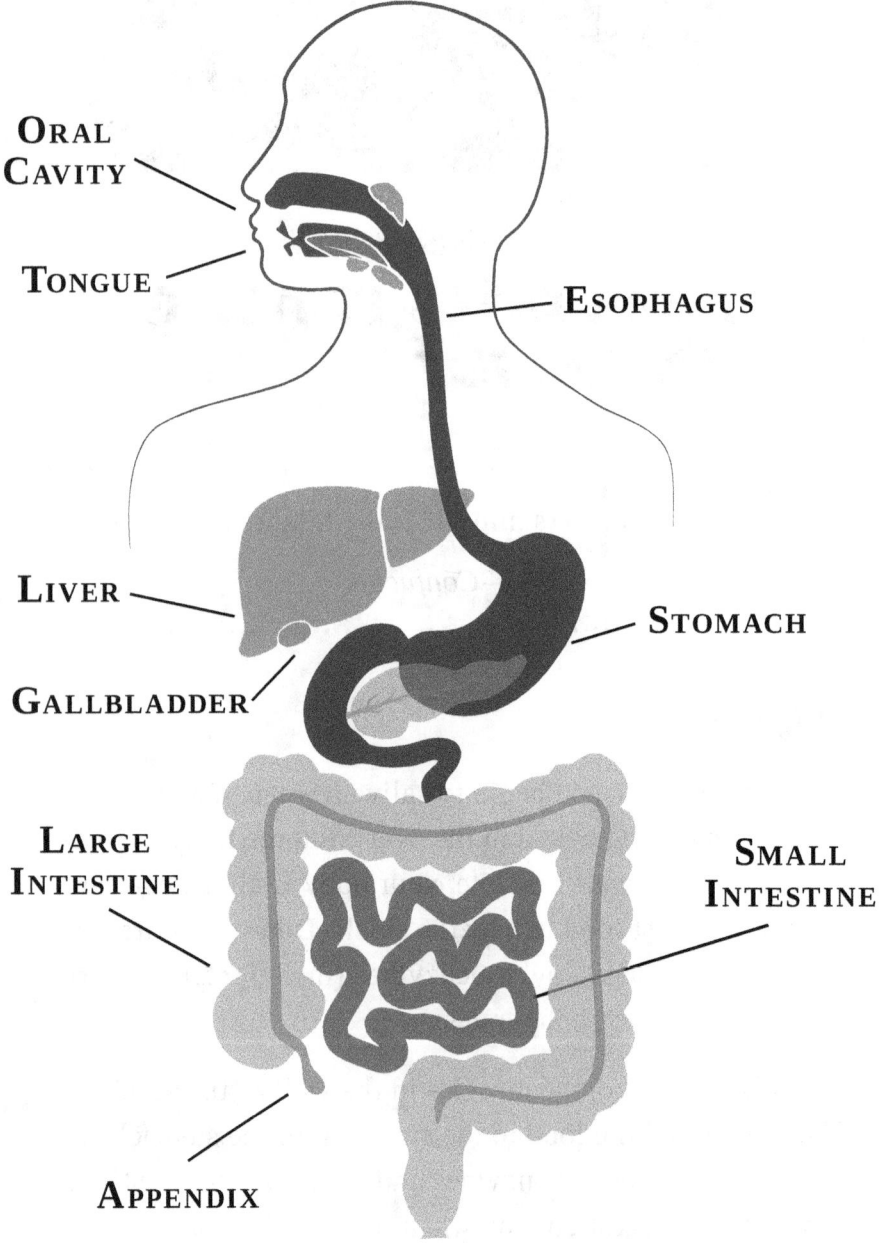

ORAL CAVITY

TONGUE

ESOPHAGUS

LIVER

STOMACH

GALLBLADDER

LARGE INTESTINE

SMALL INTESTINE

APPENDIX

The small intestine is made up of the duodenum, the jejunum and the ileum. When food enters the first part (the duodenum), the pancreas releases enzymes to break down the protein, fat and carbs. The gall bladder releases bile (that was produced in the liver and stored in the gall bladder) to assist in the breakdown of fats, so that the intestines can absorb these molecules better.

As the bile and pancreatic juices and other juices from the small intestine continue to digest the food, it passes through the jejunum (still digesting) to the ileum, where most of the nutrients are absorbed.

The waste products that remain enter the large intestine, where, if our body is functioning normally, will then expel it through the stool.

This is the simplest way to understand digestion.

Gut Microbiome

Our bodies are made up of approximately 100 trillion microbes and of these, there are estimated to be 39 trillion bacteria in the body. This includes a combination of healthy and not so healthy bacteria (or as some would say, opportunistic bacteria, always looking for a way to overtake the healthy community that is in our gut). The gut microbiome is a critical component of digestion.

More than 2,000 years ago, Hippocrates, sometimes known as the "Father of Medicine," said, "All disease begins in the gut." Fast-forward to what is going on today with our bodies and our health and you hear:

"I'm tired."

"I can't recover from my workouts the way I used to."

"My joints ache."

"I'm not sleeping well."

"There aren't enough hours in the day!"

"I'm eating right and taking care of myself, but I feel like crap."

"My hair is falling out."

"I'm eating less but can't lose weight!"

It goes on…and you know what? Generally, and I say "generally" because about 70 percent of our immune system lies in our guts, it boils down to the years of beatings our guts have taken—from food to stress to our mindset, to environment, to antibiotics, to toxins, to products, not to mention our hormones and what they do to our bodies as we enter peri-menopause and menopause. Gut health is critical to our overall health. When our gut is out of balance, we are at risk of a wide range of diseases, including type 2 diabetes, obesity, Crohn's, IBS, autoimmune disease, depression, dementia, autism, ADHD, cancer and more.

What you might not know is that your gut microbiome or environment can also affect your mood, your libido, and even how you perceive the world around you and how clearly you think. This happens through the vagus nerve, considered to be the superconductor highway between the gut and the brain. A dysfunctional microbiome can be connected to your headaches, anxiety, inability to concentrate, and depression. Nearly everything about our physical, mental and emotional health hinges upon the state of our microbiome.

And your gut microbiome starts way before you are even born. It begins with the expectant mother and father (his sperm has its own set of chromosomes that contribute to who you are when you are born) and how they took care of their bodies and then for the expectant mother, what she ate during her pregnancy (and what cleaning products, chemicals she was exposed to as well as the skin care she used) and how healthy her gut microbiome was. Two things determine our gut health: the intestinal microbiota, or "gut flora," and the gut barrier.

Gut Flora

The human gut contains over 400 known bacterial species; that's ten times more bacteria than all the human cells in our whole body. Gut flora establishes normal gastrointestinal function, provides protection from infection, and regulates our metabolism. I want to reiterate here that this flora also comprises more than 70 percent of our immune system. So, it's not surprising that when I see clients with everything from depression, IBS, IBD (including Crohn's) and Type 2 diabetes, to autoimmune conditions like Hashimoto's, psoriatic arthritis, rheumatoid arthritis and more, I can immediately link it to the possibility that they have gut flora issues.

Gut Barrier

One of the most important functions of our gut is to keep foreign substances from entering the body. But when the intestinal barrier becomes permeable, as it commonly does in "leaky gut syndrome," large protein molecules get into the bloodstream, causing the body to mount an immune response to attack them. Studies show that the repeating pattern of this process breaks down the intestinal barrier to a point that may invite autoimmune disease.

Ever had "butterflies" in your stomach? Or a "gut feeling" about something? These are terms we have used for years, but did you realize those sensations are signals from your second brain? Hidden in the walls of our digestive system is a way to understand the intimate relationship between our gut and our brain.

Our vagus nerve, the longest of our twelve cranial nerves, runs as a main channel between our abdomen (our enteric or intestinal nervous system) and our brain stem (our central nervous system). The vagus is involved in many processes in the body that don't necessarily require thought—functions like heart rate and digestion. At the same time, the bacteria in the gut directly affects the function of the cells along the vagus nerve, and some of the gut's nerve cells and microbes release neurotransmitters that "communicate" with the brain.

LEAKY GUT SYNDROME TRIGGERS

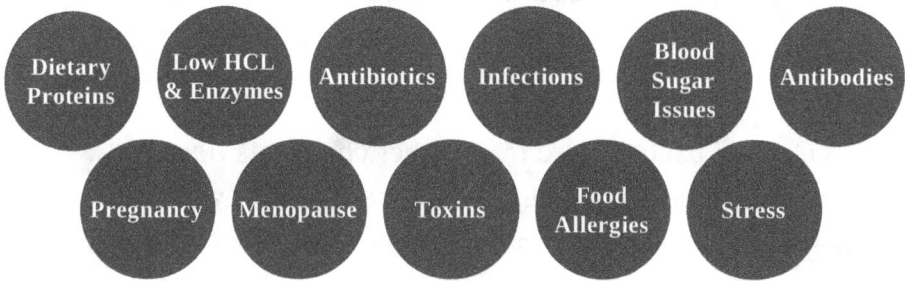

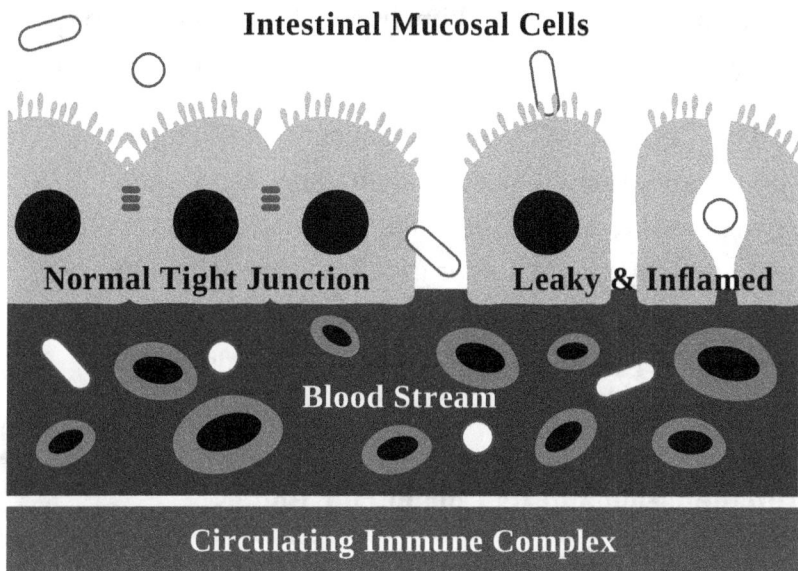

Those gut neurons and their communicative ability are why many scientists call the gut the "second brain." While gut neurons regulate muscle function, immune cells, and hormones, they also make an estimated 80 to 90 percent of the "feel-good" neurotransmitter, serotonin and melatonin (your sleep hormone). Serotonin helps regulate appetite, mood, sleep, and relaxation. This may be why, for some people, taking antidepressants may not be enough, and a change in diet needs to be considered.

Our gut bacteria also make other chemicals like the amino acid GABA, which normalizes brain waves and helps get our nervous system back to steady after it's been excited by stress. (Some foods that help increase GABA are fermented foods like kimchi and sauerkraut, almonds, walnuts, halibut, broccoli, and spinach, just to name a few.)

This fascinating brain-gut connection is a major component of how I have come to understand what my clients need to achieve optimal health. The process starts with making sure that your gut is full of healthy bacteria, which in turn has the potential not only to regulate your moods, but also, play a role in development of many diseases.

Inflammation and Its Role in Our Bodies

Did you ever get a cut? Bang into a piece of furniture or stub your toe? Your body responds to the injury and you may feel pain, swelling, redness. This is considered acute inflammation and is part of your body's defense mechanism as it reacts to help in the healing process. Usually it is short term, days, weeks, maybe a few months.

The other type of inflammation is chronic inflammation, which may last months, years, or decades. Here, the body is trying to repair and overcome damage that we might not even be aware of…yet. It occurs when a physical factor triggers an immune reaction. It could be pathogens, exposure to chemicals, acidic foods that may not agree with us. The thing with chronic inflammation is that we don't always pay attention to the signs, which is why it is so important to scan your body and *get connected* to what your symptoms are. Even something that seems benign like eczema is your body's way of talking to you. Whether it's aches and pains, rosacea, a harmless virus or something else, when left unchecked, inflammation can lead to leaky gut and disease.

Autoimmune Disease

Imagine this: One in five Americans, about 50 million people, have an autoimmune disease (AD). There are over 80 types of autoimmune diseases, affecting different parts of the body. These include conditions such as Lupus, Rheumatoid Arthritis, and Multiple Sclerosis, which occur when the immune system begins attacking the body's own organs, tissues, and cells.

What does that even mean? Why would your body attack itself?

I listened to a lot of great speakers recently at a functional nutrition conference, including Dr. Tom O'Brady, who provided what I thought was a perfect metaphor for understanding our immune system and autoimmunity. Let's consider your immune system as the Armed Forces. There's the Army, the Air Force, Navy, etc. In our bodies, let's refer to them as IgA, IgE, IgG, etc. These are the different branches of the armed forces (antibodies) in your body, and they exist to protect you. (When allergists do a skin prick test, they're looking for an IgE reaction from the triggering substance.)

If something comes into your body that doesn't belong there, your immune system fires a bullet (called a cytokine) to destroy the invader. That's your immune system trying to protect itself. What happens though is that the immune system gets confused by what's a threatening invader and what isn't. It starts attacking itself and its own tissues, like the thyroid, brain, heart, and bones. Why? Anything from the outside world coming inside us, whether it's food, the air we breathe, bugs in the water, or self-care and cleaning products, alerts your immune system to stand guard and fire off bullets to protect you. Those bullets, however, can cause collateral damage around the area. It's like a bomb hitting a target. It gets the target, but shrapnel flies everywhere, wreaking havoc.

When your cells get damaged, your body makes antibodies to get rid of the damage. The human body has an amazing capacity to heal itself. But if it's constantly killing off these invaders faster than it can replace them with healthy cells, its ability to heal itself weakens over time. Eventually, it reaches the point of raising the white flag and giving up.

That's when you've reached the tipping point. That's when you start to experience common symptoms: joint pain, abdominal pain or digestive issues, skin problems, and fatigue, for example. If you don't know why any of this is happening, you likely chalk it up to getting older or working too hard or not getting enough sleep.

What you don't know is that this has been going on in your body for *years* before you started experiencing any symptoms.

Sadly, autoimmune disease (AD) is being diagnosed more frequently than ever these days. While there was a time when it was a bit of a mystery as to what exactly was causing autoimmune issues, current research is pointing to the role gut bacteria plays in their development, as well as the liver's ability to detox properly. (More about the liver later).

When your microbiome is in great shape, your digestion works well, and you are getting and absorbing the proper nutrients. But if it's thrown off—which can happen due to anything ranging from a poor diet to medications like antibiotics to chronic stress, or even a bout of the stomach flu—some undigested toxins and unfriendly bacteria can stray from your GI tract, causing inflammation throughout your body, and in time, autoimmune disease.

It's not just about what you eat. There are also environmental factors like stress, anxiety, lack of sleep, and pollutants, cleaning products and skin care products, which also affect gut composition and the skin microbiome.

One example that gets overlooked: eczema. Eczema, also known as atopic dermatitis, is a persistent inflammation of the skin, which affects up to 17 percent of children and about six percent of adults in the US (close to 15 million Americans). While there are varying severities of eczema, they are all characterized by an extreme and sometimes painful itch that can make it difficult to focus on everyday activities and to get quality sleep.

While conventional medical views don't really seem to pinpoint a cause for eczema, the functional medicine look is clear: It is an external symptom of what is going on inside the body, as documented in 2018, in the co-authored piece, "Microbiome in the Gut-Skin Axis in Atopic Dermatitis" featured in *Allergy Asthma Immunol Res*. The underlying cause of eczema as likely to be a malfunctioning immune system. Also, if you have eczema, your chances of having asthma or seasonal allergies, also caused by inflammation and an overactive immune system response, are very high.

To review:

When your digestion isn't working optimally, a few things happen. First, your nutrient absorption is minimized, which affects the function of every system in your body. Next, poor digestion causes undigested food particles to accumulate in your GI tract, which attracts unhealthy gut bacteria to ferment there, encouraging the growth of bad bacteria in your system to outnumber the healthy gut microbes—the key communicators between your gut and brain.

All this can lead to inflammatory conditions like leaky gut syndrome, irritable bowel syndrome (IBS), irritable bowel disease (IBD, Crohn's), or SIBO (small intestine bacterial overgrowth), which all prevent gut microbes from functioning and communicating properly.

Note: American College of Gastroenterology estimates that approximately 10-15% of adults suffer from IBS symptoms, but only 5-7% have been diagnosed Is it because we all think gas, bloating and constipation (or diarrhea) are normal? Well, it's not! That's another sign your body is telling you that something is not right.

You may think, well, I've had this for as long as I can remember and it's just my body...think again.

Next, this "gut data" is sent to your brain to notify your body that your digestive tract is in trouble. At this point, this information is taking a neural pathway to reach your brain and the response is: depressive-like behaviors, anxiety, panic, mood swings, and irritability. In fact, studies by neurologists on "gut-brain axis" in 2016 point to irritable bowel syndrome as a gut-brain disorder, where depression, anxiety, and obesity are frequently seen in patients with IBS.

Can you start to see the importance of understanding? When you get what is going on, it's an opportunity to shift the focus on what you can do and to also understand that while you may have done things differently before, be kind to yourself and tell yourself that it's okay. This didn't occur overnight. It took years. You didn't know what you didn't know (unconsciously incompetent) but now that you do (consciously incompetent), you have a choice.

Before we get to another activity for you to complete, I want to touch on a few other items.

Other Hormones and Your Gut

While this book isn't about hormones (and there are plenty of great resources available), there are a few I want to share as it relates to gut health. Our body's endocrine system produces more than fifty hormones, many of which have a major impact on our health and wellbeing, and most seem to have a relationship with our gut microbiota. Let's look at some of the top ones:

- *Cortisol* (made in the adrenal glands) is a hormone released during times of stress. Too much of it can wreck our sense of calm and peace. Research shows we can work to reduce levels of cortisol in the body by balancing our gut bacteria.

- *Estrogen* is primarily a female hormone, but men do have small amounts. The levels of this hormone are affected by our digestion—so supporting a balanced gut microbiota helps our body to keep excess estrogen out of circulation.

- *Insulin* is secreted by the pancreas and allows cells to absorb blood glucose, which in turn, is used for energy. Studies show that probiotic balance in the gut can support healthy insulin levels warding off metabolic diseases.

- *Leptin* is made by our fat cells and signals the brain when it is time to stop eating. A healthy gut can help our brain from becoming resistant to that message, helping us to maintain a healthy weight.

- *Grehlin* (the hunger hormone) is produced mainly in the gut and travels through your bloodstream to your brain, where it tells it that it is hungry. When you start a diet and restrict too many calories, this hunger hormone kicks in because your body is trying to protect you from starvation mode. Over time, the constant dieting lowers your metabolic rate, making it harder to lose weight and keep it off.

Gut Health and Aging

A common complaint I hear from some of my older patients (and even some younger ones) is that they are experiencing joint pain and stiffness and need to find relief. While it is true that as we age and the connective tissue and cartilage that cushion our joints thins and wears down, we can feel pain and inflammation; what most don't realize is that part of the equation is related to gut health, not just the wear and tear on joints over time or aging.

What Is Arthritis?

Arthritis is the term commonly used to describe an array of about 200 conditions that affect joints, the tissues that surround the joints, and other connective tissue. A survey conducted by CDC between 2013-2015 estimated that 22.7% (54.4 million) of adults had doctor diagnosed arthritis. By the year 2040, an estimated 78.4 million (25.9% of the projected total adult population) adults (18 years and older) will have doctor-diagnosed arthritis. Two-thirds of those with arthritis will be women.

Other studies show that two common kinds of arthritis, osteoarthritis and rheumatoid arthritis, can be helped through diet and balancing the gut microbiome. While it is important to eat a balanced diet and avoid refined, processed foods to help maintain a healthy weight and control overall inflammation, unless your gut health is in balance, those efforts may fall short of helping you get the relief you are seeking from pain.

In 2013, research funded by NIH's National Institute of Arthritis and Musculoskeletal and Skin Diseases, National Institute of Allergy and Infectious Diseases, and National Human Genome Research Institute linked the gut microbiome to rheumatoid arthritis, which is a debilitating, autoimmune disease. Results appeared in *eLife*, and I have to tell you that the information begs the question: Can our gut heal our joints? A growing number of researchers are finding that it may be possible.

Pioneering research has been done by Dr. Jose Scher, a rheumatologist at New York University Langone Medical Center. Scher has been studying the connection between intestinal bugs and arthritis and in two particular studies, found that people with rheumatoid arthritis were much more likely to have a bug called *Prevotella copri* in their intestines than people that did not have the disease.

In a different study, Scher found that patients with psoriatic arthritis, another kind of autoimmune joint disease, had significantly lower levels of other types of intestinal bacteria.

Also, in the forefront of researching the gut microbiome connection to joint pain and inflammation is widely respected microbiome expert Dr. Martin Blaser of NYU, who believes our unhealthy diets full of processed foods and chemicals, the overuse of antibiotics, and a decrease in contact with the microbe-packed natural world of animals and plants have changed our microbiome significantly over the past century, and especially over the past fifty years.

Scher and Blaser are both looking into a range of potential strategies to use bacteria as medicine for immune disorders and how to modify the microbiome through dietary changes that include having more wild fish, olive oil and vegetables and low in meat and saturated fat that in turn can help reduce arthritic inflammation.

Your Liver

I have to give notable mention to the liver due to its symbiotic relationship with the gut.

The liver is truly unique. It is the only organ in the body that can regenerate itself. Kinda cool, right? The liver does not get much attention until we talk about alcoholism and then automatically think *cirrhosis of the liver* or *fatty liver.* It's one of those supporting actors in the play called life, but really, it does have a leading role! One of the many jobs that the liver has is to produce bile that helps digest fats and some vitamins. Whatever needs to be used is transported to the small intestine and the rest gets stored in the gallbladder. The liver also stores glycogen, which is used as a buffer if blood glucose levels decrease.

The liver also metabolizes fats, proteins and carbohydrates, and guess what? Because it cares about our bodies so much, it will hold toxins there just to protect our bodies. *Toxins, detox.* Now, I get why people detox (mentioned later), but the question is, shouldn't I take care of my liver regularly and not just once in a while? Of course. And part of learning what that means to you is to understand that while we can't exactly control the air we breathe or the environment we live in, we can control what we eat, what skin care products we use, what cleaning supplies and detergents we use, what pots and pans we cook with, and what type of water we drink.

Think of the liver as a swimming pool. The pool contains filters to get rid of the leaves and dirt and other organic material that lands in the water. When the filter isn't working, the leaves and other items just float around. Over time, if the filter isn't fixed, the pool fills up and the material has nowhere to go. It sits. Dirt accumulates at the bottom of the pool. No one wants to go swimming because they can't see the bottom of what was once clear water. Imagine that this is the liver and instead of the debris, your liver starts to become sluggish (and may exacerbate your symptoms).

Start your day with a glass of room temperature lemon (or lime) water in the morning. This helps to kickstart the digestive system ready for the day and helps cleanse the liver. Use fresh lemon, lemon balm or organic essential lemon oil. Daily. Simple ways to get started and express love for your liver are adding fennel, parsley, cilantro, celery, cucumber, and/or tarragon.

Speaking of love (your liver and your whole body), what we say to ourselves is so important. Do you know anyone who has ever been bullied or has done the bullying? Imagine how the words feel to the person. They're hurtful, and unfortunately, in too many instances, teenagers have committed suicide as a result of bullying (cyber and otherwise). The words that we hear, whether they are from other people or ourselves, has a great impact on our mental, emotional and physical state. You've heard the expression, "Words can cut like a knife." They leave scars if they are negative and over time, if we hear the same messages repeatedly, it can impact our health. The reverse is true as well. Think of a time when you've been complimented or given words of encouragement. How did that make you feel?

In 1848, German professor Gustav Fechner published the book, *Nanna (Soul-life of Plants),* stating that plants benefit from human conversation. While there isn't a lot of research in this area, IKEA, the DIY furniture retailer, conducted a bullying experiment on plants in 2018 in the United Arab Emirates. They placed two identical plants near each other and for thirty days, invited students to compliment one plant and bully the other. After thirty days, the plant that was given the compliments was healthy and thriving and the one that was bullied, was wilted.

While this isn't exactly scientific, some theorize that it is the vibration of sound that elicited the responses in the plants. Regardless, what's important and the reason I share this is because again, being healthy is more than just the foods we eat. Words can be equally powerful. They can help us thrive or they can be toxic to our bodies. Being mindful of not only the words you choose to use in conversation but also, the words you choose to say to yourself ("I can't believe how stupid I am", or "I have a dumb question to ask"). Realize that the repetitive nature of the words can have a huge impact on all aspects of your health. Find compassion for self.

WRITING EXERCISE
DIGEST AND DISCOVER

Look back at your notes, at all the items you checked off in the Getting Connected section and think about your life. Maybe you had ear infections growing up and were on antibiotics frequently. Who knew back then how antibiotics kill off not only the bad bacteria but also, the good. Continue to make connections and soon, I'll give you many ideas of what action steps you can take that work for *you*!

THE G.U.T. METHOD®

Get connected to your symptoms,
what you're thinking, how you're feeling.

CHAPTER *10*

GUT REACTIONS

....

"Dear Stress, I would like a divorce.
Please understand it is not you, it is me."

—*Thomas E. Rojo Aubrey*

....

Approximately 40 million adults in the U.S age 18+ suffer from anxiety disorders, and anxiety disorder is considered the most common mental illness in the U.S. It is thought that it develops from a complex set of factors, which include genetics, life events, and of course, brain chemistry and gut imbalance.

The main difference between anxiety and stress is that stress is the reaction to a threatening situation (or what is perceived to be a threat) and anxiety is a reaction to stress. You may have heard of the fight or flight response where when a person experiences or even perceives a stressful event, the body reacts by releasing hormones that prepare your body to fight or run away.

What is the real effect of stress on our gut? Deadline after deadline to get it all done at work. Home projects piling up and not enough time to get it done. Marital issues, finances, taking care of ailing parents, etc. Daily stresses that shorten our breath and make our heart race. Even if we are eating well, exercising and doing everything right, studies show that most stressful life events could be setting us up for several digestive conditions like inflammatory bowel disease like Crohn's disease, irritable bowel syndrome, gastroesophageal reflux or GERD and stomach ulcers. In all of these, it is clear that stress affects both the systemic and gastrointestinal immune and inflammatory responses in our bodies.

One client, Carly, who was under so much stress at her job, was constantly getting sick. Looking at her on the outside, she is tall, slim, and no one would suspect that her body was falling apart. However, she was often fatigued, light-headed and depressed. Endless appointments with doctors and specialists led her to be diagnosed with narcolepsy and chronic insomnia and soon her life was controlled by medications. When we started working together, she thought she was eating healthy and looked it on the outside. She slowly started connecting how her symptoms—the stress at work, what she thought were healthy food options (including sandwiches with processed meat)—and realized that her immune system had taken such a beating. Once she analyzed her symptoms (she was a banker, after all), she was able to understand how over time, it had taken its toll on her body and her life. Carly was eventually able to stop all her medications and bring her body, her mind and her sanity back into balance. Her favorite way to decompress was breathing, which for her, led to yoga and to becoming a certified yoga instructor!

Life or Death, With Every Breath

I toyed with where to place this section because technically, it represents action. But it felt right to place it here especially after sharing Carly's story. Breathing is one of the very first things we do when we are born and the last thing we do before we die, but how much attention do we really pay to it? You probably don't think twice about your breathing patterns most of the time because they are so automatic. Imagine this though; over the course of a day, adults and older children usually breathe 17,000-30,000 breaths per day—or more! The bottom line is we can stay alive for long periods of time without eating, drinking or sleeping, but not very long without breathing.

Breathing: Physical and Metaphysical

Breathing is physically important for two main reasons: It supplies our bodies and organs with oxygen, which is vital for survival. Interestingly, that oxygen cannot be stored and must be replenished continuously and steadily, so it is important to know how to breathe properly. It helps us get rid of waste products and toxins from the body some of which we have created and through improper breathing can easily stagnate in our bodies and damage our vital functions.

On a metaphysical level, we've known for ages from yoga practitioners that proper breathing circulates *prana* or life force energy in our bodies, connecting us to our battery or solar plexus. This is why in yoga there are several breathing techniques known as pranayama that help set this energy in motion to revitalize the body and mind.

Slow Breathing

The key to beginning the process of proper breathing is to slow it down, in general. Unfortunately, most of us take short breaths and use only a small portion— about a third of our lung capacity when breathing. We also tend to breathe into the upper chest with hunched shoulders, leading to a lack of oxygen and tension in the upper back and the neck. Some other signs of improper breathing include:

- Holding the breath at times

- Feeling the need for a long breath

- Running out of breath when we are moving faster

Breathing and the Mind

Breathing links body and mind, both need oxygen to function well. It also moves energy in our body. By learning how to breathe well, we can be in better control of our emotions and fears and keep a clear and sharp mind. Irregular breathing can make our minds nervous, agitated, and anxious. If our breathing is deep, slow, and regular then our mind will more likely be calmer.

Breathing for Stress Relief

One of the most potent effects of breathing properly is how it can counteract the adverse effects of stress including hypertension, anxiety, insomnia and aging. The American Psychological Association has repeatedly published surveys correlating stress levels to feelings of being unhealthy. Stress can trigger an instantaneous sequence of hormonal changes and physiological responses, which over time, can take a toll on our body.

One of my favorite ways to decrease stress is a breathing exercise that doesn't require you to meditate. I touched on this earlier for getting connected, but here is the breathing exercise in-depth, using your five senses, counteracting the stress response through observing the breath:

- Sit quietly on a sofa or comfortable chair, with your legs uncrossed, touching the floor, your head in a comfortable position with eyes closed and your hands sitting loosely on your lap.

- Deeply relax all your muscles, beginning at your feet and up to your face. Soften your jaw. Let your hands sit loosely on your lap.

- Breathe in through your nose and out through your mouth. Become aware of your breathing. No judgment. Just notice. Breathe easily and naturally.

- As you sit breathing, bring your attention to your senses. Let's start with touch. With each breath, notice the clothes on your body. What do they feel like? Soft? Itchy? Comfortable? What about the chair or sofa? Just notice how you feel sitting there.

- Next, let's go to your sense of hearing. Listen to what feels close by. Maybe it's the hum of the air conditioner; maybe it's a car honking outside. Notice what you hear in the distance. Maybe it's voices. Again, we're just noticing here. No judgment. No right or wrong. It's just sound passing through our ear canal.

- Keep breathing and bring your attention to your nose. What do you smell? Maybe nothing, maybe perfume or room freshener. Just breathe through it and notice it.

- Next, even though your eyes will be closed for this breathing exercise, you may still see shapes and shades of color. Notice them as you keep breathing.

- Now, think about taste. As you breathe in and out through your nose (or in through your nose and out through your mouth), notice if you feel anything in your mouth. Maybe you just ate a piece of salmon and you not only smell it but you taste it in your mouth, or maybe your mouth feels dry. Again, just notice.

- With each breath, as you bring yourself to pay attention to your senses, your body starts to relax.

- You can do this for 5 minutes or longer!

Remember my client, the lawyer? At the end of this exercise, when I asked how she felt, she said she was more tired than before the exercise. We talked about how stressed she was and how her body was on such high alert, that just breathing through her senses for 5 minutes, exhausted her. I wasn't surprised, given the intensity of her day. We discussed when she could practice this so that she would feel relaxed and not exhausted, and over time, her ability to focus on breathing helped her during the day without exhausting her.

Learning to breathe properly isn't hard to do. You just need to find the time for yourself to bring it in to your life so it can become a habit, much like brushing your teeth. There are many other types of breathing exercises that you can incorporate. Some favorite ones of my clients can be found on YouTube, including the 4, 7, 8 breathing technique where you breathe in through your nose for a count of 4, hold for a count of 7 and breathe out through your moth for a count of 8.

Another method is square breathing. With this method, you use your thumb and ring finger of one hand. Press your thumb on one nostril and breathe in through your other nostril for a count of 4. Hold for a count of 4. Then switch nostrils and use your ring finger to press the other nostril and breathe out through the first nostril for a count of 4. Hold your breath again for a count of 4 and keep cycling. This can also be found on YouTube. The benefits of conscious breathing are well worth incorporating into your daily life. Even a little practice goes a long way and can be life-changing.

Sleep and Your Gut

It's no secret that if you're not getting quality sleep, your mental and physical health will be compromised. Studies now show that gut microbiota imbalances can interfere with our sleep quality and our very important circadian rhythm (sleep-wake cycle).

There is also emerging evidence that circadian rhythms regulate the gut immune response and can play a role in sleep disturbances, obesity, metabolic and inflammatory disease, and mood disorders. This is particularly important for shift workers and others who experience regular changes to their sleep/wake patterns.

Just like we need the neurotransmitter serotonin to ward off depression and other health issues, we need melatonin, the "sleep" hormone, in order to ward off insomnia and allow our bodies to rest and digest. Melatonin signals the body when it is time to rest, but our gut microbiota (where a good percentage of melatonin is produced), needs to support the conversion of tryptophan to serotonin to melatonin. Without that support, we are set up to experience both down moods as well as sleepless nights.

Our Ecstatic, Dramatic Lives: The Truth About Emotions

Confession: I drew you to breathing exercises before addressing emotions because I figured you would need the spacious breath in order to continue here!

As we continue to peel back the layers of your gut and its connection to mental health, I want to continue with the emotional side. I'm not a psychologist, but I am fascinated with how our brains work. I love reading and learning about neuroplasticity and the power we have to change our brains, so what I'm sharing with you is my own understanding of what this means and how we can use our minds to our advantage in our understanding of our actions.

Our conscious mind is our awareness. It's responsible for our logical thinking. If I asked you what one plus one equals, you'd say two. When the alarm goes off, you wake up. When the teakettle whistles, you turn the burner off.

The subconscious mind is responsible for your involuntary actions like breathing. It is responsible for your emotions and is also where your beliefs and memories are stored. That's why just repeating affirmations doesn't generally work. If your belief system is subconscious but you're consciously stating affirmations, your subconscious is filtering those thoughts. This is where it gets complicated, but where it is also very exciting. Once you become aware of your habits and your thoughts, you can start asking yourself questions to debunk your own thinking.

As for the unconscious mind, Freudian theory is that it is a reservoir of feelings, thoughts and memories that are outside the conscious mind, and that many of those are our feelings of pain, anxiety and /or conflict. Ah...interesting. If it's unconscious and it's feelings of pain, anxiety and/or conflict, how do we ever become aware of it to do anything about it?

Unconsciously Incompetent

You don't know what you don't know. So, it's up to you to decide what you want to explore...and if you need help doing so, or not. Here's the thing. There is no right or wrong. There is only what is. Or you can look at it from Yoda's point of view: The scene from "Star Wars" where Luke has already given up before he even tried because he doubts his own abilities. Yoda tells him he must unlearn what he has learned. Luke says he'll try and Yoda says, "No! Try not. Do. Or do not. There is no try."

When I was married, my life looked perfect on paper. Great husband. Kids. House in the suburbs, a pool in our backyard, vacations, sleep-away camp for the kids every summer. Smiles on our faces. Perfect on the outside!

I remember our last trip as a family. We went on a Club Med ski vacation to a family resort at Copper Mountain in Colorado. We settled in our first day, rented skis, became familiar with the resort and went to bed early. We had flown in from New York and the time change and altitude had taken its toll.

The first morning, the kids went off to the kids' camp and the adults were tested to see which group they would join for group ski lessons. My former husband was a much better skier than me, so we were put into separate groups.

The weather was beautiful. Clear skies, mid-30s, and no wind. Perfect. The only noise you heard besides our voices was the swish of the snow as the skiers glided past us.My group was a mix of men and women mostly in the same age range and we got to know each other during the course of the week.

Around our third or fourth day in, I was taking the chairlift up with a couple of the guys and they started talking about divorce. At that time, I knew I was unhappy, that something was off in my life and my marriage, but kept thinking it was me, that this was life, that I had chosen this path, and never considered that it was us, so the word, *divorce*, was a foreign concept to me. My friends were all married. I was raised to believe that you get married for better or worse, in good times and bad, 'til death do you part and that you can fix it, whatever that meant.

Here, on this beautiful day, these two guys were talking about divorce and how they knew so many couples who weren't happy and considering separating.

My first reaction (to myself) was, I admit, judgmental. Yeah, so what? Life isn't a bowl of cherries and sometimes you're not happy. Deal with it. At that point, I tuned out the conversation. But throughout the course of that week, the word, divorce, kept popping into my head. I started asking myself what does even mean? Divorce. Did you fail if you got divorced? And then I asked myself, *how do you know if you should get divorced?*

Well, the answer would ultimately come a year and a half later, while mindlessly flipping through the channels on TV. I came upon "The Dr, Phil Show," which, to be honest, is not my cup of tea. Something stopped me from changing the channels though. There were two couples sitting across from him. At the exact moment that I tuned into that station, he was telling one of the couples that they had tried everything, turned over every stone, in an attempt to work on their marriage, but it was obvious that they had completely grown apart and would be better off getting divorced than staying in an unhappy marriage, and that eventually, the kids would understand.

What? Did I just hear that correctly? I had turned over every stone. I had tried everything I could think of. Did I have this all wrong? Is divorce something I can do? I had planned almost everything in my life. Wasn't that what I was supposed to do? Was something wrong with me? Can I get divorced? What would everyone think? And how embarrassing to think I'd failed. Failing wasn't an option. Yet, a little voice started to wonder. There was a crack.

That was over fifteen years ago. Now, I can easily see how I had been eating my emotions, both literally and emotionally, and how that stress and energy manifested in my body, as well as the foods I was eating that weren't right for my body, the self-shame I was feeling, the inadequacy of not being good enough, the symptoms I had been experiencing. Now, opportunities were presenting themselves that made me realize I had to pay attention because where before I didn't think I had a choice, I was waking up to the fact that I did. I needed to be honest with myself and be willing to own my actions and hold myself accountable. I needed to look inward, do some deep soul searching and figure out what I wanted. I needed to understand how to unwrap it all. And for me, it started with therapy. First private therapy, then Landmark Education, then Tony Robbins, Dr. Bruce Lipton, Joe Dispenza and the dozens of books I read to help me rewire my brain. To help me connect the dots. To help me understand that just because I had lived my life one way didn't mean I couldn't change it. That being said, please note that this was my journey. I'm not in any way implying or telling you that divorce is what you need. And honestly, while I was scared and experienced anxiety and panic attacks during the process because my life as I knew it, as I had planned it had gone off the cliff, I wouldn't change anything about my life or my choices because had I not made these choices, I wouldn't have the gift of my three children. They're my why for everything that I do. I also would not be who I am today. Who knows how I would have handled my son's diagnosis or if I would have gone to grad school or found my passion; and who knows if this book would ever have been written? I do believe that everything happens for a reason and when the same sign keeps knocking at your door, you have to pause and take notice, because if you don't, trust me, the universe will find a way to get to you!

By understanding that your unconscious needs to be awakened in order for you to start reframing your thoughts, you'll then be able to shift the conversation, whether it's with yourself or with others. A way to start is to first become aware of your thoughts: the ones you think and the ones you share.

When my twins were graduating college, my older son, Evan, and I were in the car driving from one college to the other. Murphy's Law would have them graduate not just the same weekend, but the same day! Many tears were shed, mostly mine, as we had to divide and conquer. The one saving grace was that at least their colleges were a three-hour drive from each other, so we were able to celebrate as a family the next day. On this drive, Evan and I were talking about his sister Nicki's desire to become a music therapist.

"Too bad no one told her she won't be making a lot of money as a music therapist," said Evan.

I paused. "What makes you say that?"

"Music therapists don't make a lot of money."

"Oh? Where did you hear that?"

My son's turn to pause. "Hmm. I don't know."

"Then is it true? Is that what you believe?"

Another pause. This time a lengthy one. My kids know that when I start asking these types of questions, they need to think. Yes, I used to get the eye rolling sometimes. The beauty is that our conversations are non-judgmental; they're about getting to our truths and in that moment, my son's perception about that comment shifted.

I remember another instance back when my daughter was in middle school. She was playing softball and hit a line drive down center. As she slid into first base, she hit her foot on the side of the base and heard a noise. She had fractured her ankle. She needed surgery and had pins put in. Not fun to be in a cast right before the middle school prom!

When I took Nicki to PT, on the first visit, the guy said, "You won't heal 100%, but we'll get almost as good as new." I was upset.

"How do you know that?" I asked him.

His response: "I've seen this so many times and it's just what happens." I didn't respond, but when we left, I looked at my daughter and I said, "Don't believe a word he says. He doesn't know your body. I believe you are going to heal, and I want you to believe it also." I was so annoyed. Did he think he was God? Did he have a crystal ball? P.S. My daughter did heal 100%. She's better than ever. She skis, snowboards and hikes, and is not limited in any way from that injury. What you believe is central to your health.

WRITING EXERCISE
DIGEST AND DISCOVER

We talked about how we can put limiting beliefs on ourselves and if we speak what we think our truth is, it may plant a seed for others to start thinking the same thing. Close your eyes and observe your thoughts. What are you saying to yourself? Is it true? Why do you believe that? Where did it come from? Write without judgment, without editing. Then ask 'what if' questions. What if it's not true that I have to diet? What if there is another way? What if I don't weigh myself and go by how my clothes feel on me?

_____

_____

_____

_____

_____

_____

_____

_____

_____

_____

_____

_____

_____

_____

_____

_____

You have to dissect beliefs to find the truth, between the facts of what happened as an occurrence and the story you told yourself. This takes time. By dissecting the conversations, you are having with yourself, you can start figuring out and understanding where your language, the words you use, your expectations and beliefs came from. Then, you can start paying attention and writing it down. This is all part of shifting your perspective. Your point of view is in your control. No matter what stories you told yourself in the past, NOW is the time to ask yourself: Does this serve me? If it's not true and it doesn't serve, now is the time to create a shift, create a new perspective that makes you feel like a warrior instead of a victim.

First, identify what is bothering you physically, emotionally, or mentally. Pick one item that seems to recur. Did something trigger it?

Maybe it occurs when you think about a stressful situation. Maybe it gets triggered when someone says something to you. Words are so important and if not used properly can become weapons without our even realizing it.

Start noticing the correlation. Write it down and observe when it happens and how often. Once you do that, you can start connecting your own dots. Keep repeating the question to see how deep to the root you can get and journal what is coming up for you.

_____

_____

_____

_____

_____

_____

_____

_____

_____

_____

My client, the lawyer, can prepare and argue a case like it's no one's business. She knows what she needs to do because she learned how. Since we started working together, she's gone down two pant sizes, but she doesn't feel that's enough. She has in her mind the number she wants to see on the scale when she goes to her doctor, and she gets angry at herself when she doesn't see that number.

Here are a few things she says to herself:

• Food is not my friend.

- Why is losing weight so hard for me?

- I'm not eating much, but the scale hasn't budged since I weighed myself the week after starting detox.

- This is so frustrating.

- Nothing is working, and it's very upsetting.

- CALM. DOWN. PLEASE!

- JUST RELAX.

Sound familiar? I asked her to keep track every day. I asked her to pay attention to what she was saying to herself and how often throughout the day she was doing so. I didn't ask her to do anything about it except to pay attention, write it down, and notice the time. We spoke halfway through the week. The first few days, she was shocked at how often she had these thoughts and how she had them throughout the day. She didn't like what she was reading. Great! Now that she was aware, now that she was conscious and connected, she could start understanding how this was affecting her and take action.

By the middle of the second week, for two days in a row, she was happy to report that she had no negative self-talk.

Your body is really this perfect antenna that is receptive to navigating through the ups and downs. You wouldn't tune into FM radio when you want to listen to the ball game on AM radio. It's a different frequency, and you won't get the game. All you'll get is noise that you don't want to hear because you're not tuned into the right frequency.

If you don't pay attention to it, trust me, the screams will be deafening, until you end up at the doctor's office wondering what happened.

Don't get me wrong. Doctors are awesome. They save lives. But we have to be our own health advocates in all senses of the word, even with our practitioners. If there's something that doesn't sit right, don't just believe it because they're the expert. Challenge them but do so with kindness. Come to your appointment with a list of questions that you want answers to. Share your journal with them so that they can understand what's going on with you. *This is a collaboration.* Remember that your doctor is in a position of serving you. If there's information that you need to share with them, don't *expect* them to read your mind and don't be embarrassed. Be honest. Everyone has similar symptoms, and you have to help each other understand one another, and what you are each saying so that you can map out the right route for *you.*

Detox and Holistic Rejuvenation

What doctors may not readily talk to you about, no matter what ailment you do or do not have, is detox. What do you think of when you hear the word detox? Liquid diet? Starve yourself? Lemon water, a little cayenne pepper and a drop of maple syrup for four days?

Tea that will get rid of belly fat?

I fell under the detox spell years ago thinking that if I cleansed my body in three or four days, I'd be fine. I'd lose weight and feel great. I'd get rid of my stomach aches and clean out (whatever that meant) my body. First off, I was miserable with this liquid diet. I had been told, wait a few days, you'll feel so much better and have more energy, and I did (temporarily) but not before I had to walk around like a zombie willing myself to stand up. Why was I putting myself through this? Why do you? Seriously, why do we do this shit to ourselves? What does it prove? A false sense of bravado and willpower?

It never occurred to me that I was eating advertisements. That I was following the herd. All I thought was that if it worked for that person it will certainly work for me. I was on auto pilot and just *knew* that this had to be the answer.

Once I went off the detox and went back to my old ways of eating, I would gain the weight back (and then some) and feel lousy again. No one ever explained what detoxing meant. It became one of those buzz words until I learned about the importance of our liver in the detoxification process and that there was a healthy way to go about this thing called *detox*. It involves adding in the right foods to support our bodies, all of which you will discover as you begin to take action.

THE G.U.T. METHOD®

Get connected to your symptoms,
what you're thinking, how you're feeling.

CHAPTER *11*

FROM STILLNESS LEAPS ACTION

....

"Life isn't about finding yourself.
Life is about creating yourself."

—*George Bernard Shaw*

....

This section is where you will put the pieces of your puzzle together. You must first decide how ready you are for your journey. Below is a list of areas for you to think about. On a scale of 1 (not sure if I'm ready for all of it but thanks for the information) to 5 (YES! I'm all in), check off where you are in each are:

	1	2	3	4	5
Implement shifts into your 'diet'					
Modify lifestyle					
Improve sleep habits					
Keep a food journal					
Practice a relaxation technique					
Engage in regular exercise					
How supportive are the key people in your life during this process					

Within your answers, you will slowly start to see how small changes in your habits and mindset can catapult you from impossible to possible, from powerless to empowered. You will look at your journey with a new perspective: This is a marathon, not a sprint and the chart above is just a gauge for you.

Transformative Actions

Babies start by taking one step. They may cry when they fall down, but it doesn't deter them. They get right back up. They don't create a story about why they fell. They pick themselves up and try again. Think of this as your rebirth. Your new body, your outlook starts today. You can walk, jog or run. I'm going to outline ideas into three sections for you to review with the goal being to pick one component from each section to be your foundation and then each week (or two, depending on the speed you choose), add an additional component.

The first section is *laying the foundation and creating awareness.*

The second section is the *food / planning* section and has a variety of components. It's not in any particular order. Again, take it at a pace that works for you. You decide where you want to start. I think the biggest reason that diets fail is because we aren't given a choice. We are told what to do, what to remove, and if you're anything like me, when someone says no, I'll do just the opposite! But when you have freedom to choose how you want to approach your lifestyle shifts, you'll be more successful.

The third section is the *mind/body* component.

Again, pick one each week so that you can create new habits slowly.

Don't let these suggestions overwhelm you. I recommend reading through them once and allow yourself to sit with them and reflect with what resonates with you most. When we get overwhelmed, it may lead to analysis paralysis and I don't want you to quit before you even start. I know. I've been there. So eager to want to do it all *now* and get the results *now* and figure it out *now*...you get the gist.

Let's start with the first section.

1. Laying the Foundation and Creating Awareness

- **Focus on your breath.** Maybe for you, it's just slowing down and breathing and being with your body and noticing what you're feeling. Maybe the breathing will help you with your stress and anxiety. You can refer back to the chapter with a few of the breathing techniques to get you started.

- **Drink more water.** While the general rule of thumb is approximately half your body weight in ounces, this will vary depending on your activity level, geographic location and time of year. As I mentioned in Chapter 8, water is essential to our existence. You can infuse it with berries, citrus, cucumber, mint or just drink it plain. You can include your unsweetened tea and coffee in this category, but sorry people, alcohol does not count!

- **Chew your food.** You're probably thinking, *really?* Yes, really. This does take practice and there will be times when you're out to dinner having fun that you'll forget! It's okay. You may even want to bring this to the dinner table as a game with your kids. Maybe you want them to try a new food. You can have your whole family take the bite and count 20-30 times until the food is mushy in your mouth and then have everyone stick out their tongues to see whose is mushiest. I know it sounds gross, but it could be a fun way to get them to try something new.

2. Food / Planning

- **Pick one meal to work on improving the quality of the food.** There's a lot of talk about removing highly allergenic foods like wheat, corn, soy, peanuts, dairy, nuts, eggs. If you have sensitivities or allergies or specific gut or health issues that you are aware of and working on, you will want to remove them promptly. You may be that person who finds it easy to eliminate foods completely right away. That's great! Or you may choose to do food sensitivity testing. *Whatever works for you.* But for many who are just starting out, it feels overwhelming to remove so many foods at once because you may not be ready and then you are setting yourself up for failure. As soon as you forget and "cheat" you start feeling guilty and the self-sabotage sets in and then you throw in the towel and give up. Instead, we're going to re-frame and have a new perspective on how you look at your choices. The key is being consistent so that you build a solid foundation that becomes integral to your lifestyle. Below are a few ideas:

  Maybe you aren't ready to give up bread but are willing to upgrade the quality of what you are buying. For example, instead of the store brand that comes in a bag with a million ingredients, you upgrade to organic bread or sprouted bread.

  Perhaps you love pasta. You can swap regular pasta for chickpea or black bean or cauliflower pasta. If you're not ready for that, opt for brown rice pasta or other type that has no wheat.

Maybe you want to start with breakfast. Instead of coffee and a bagel or a bowl of cereal with milk, try overnight oats or avocado toast. Instead of drinking a glass of juice, eat an orange.

Eat whole foods. Maybe you don't eat a lot of vegetables. Start with something as easy as making mashed cauliflower instead of mashed potatoes.

Try adding in a new vegetable this week. Think of the colors of the rainbow. Choose different vegetables and keep adding new ones. With awareness and practice, you will find ways to be creative.

Swap out dairy for non-dairy. There are quite a few options: unsweetened coconut milk, almond milk, cashew milk (you can even make your own)

Are you eating too much sugar and want to cut back? Start by looking at nutrition labels and seeing how much sugar is in a product. Make sure there is more protein and fiber (combined) than sugar. Another step is to pay attention to the added sugar in your food journal and upgrade to a food that is a healthier option (see the next idea).

- **Upgrade your snack.** Generally, if you eat three healthy meals, you may only need one snack. It depends on when you woke up or what your activity level was for the day. Snacking for some comes more from a habit than hunger. That being said, there are times when you may need a snack because you may not have had enough protein, fiber and healthy fats at your previous meal. The goal is to minimize eating processed foods. For instance, pretzels seem like such an innocuous snack. Fat free, easy to bring with you, won't spoil, what's so bad? It's all simple carbohydrates and while it may give you a quick pop of energy, your blood sugar will spike and then drop, and you'll probably still be hungry. To build a healthy power snack that will provide you with energy, satiate you, keep the brain fog at bay and keep your blood sugar balanced, consider a snack from the list below:

An organic apple sprinkled with chia seeds or ground flaxseeds. ("An apple a day helps keep the doctor away!")

Celery, almond butter and sunflower seeds.

Celery, an apple and a couple of dates.

Hummus with carrots and cucumbers.

Avocado and any green leafy vegetables.

Guacamole and carrots/broccoli/cauliflower/tomato.

How about a smoothie? Be careful here. Most smoothies are fruit and juice (or milk) and that will only spike your blood sugar. Make or purchase one with non-dairy milk, a few berries, handful of spinach, vegan protein powder (or hemp) and you may even want to add ¼ avocado or nut butter. There are so many ways to build a healthy snack.

- **Start reading nutrition labels and upgrade the foods you buy.** Shop the perimeter of the supermarket where the fresh produce lives. The center aisles belong to all that processed food that we want to minimize. That being said, when you do buy snacks, crackers, nut butters or other items, look at the labels and find one that has the fewest ingredients. If you are used to buying the national favorite peanut butter that you've seen on TV ads, look at the label and find one that has just two ingredients: nuts and sea salt. If you can't find it at the regular supermarket, there's probably an all-natural store in your neighborhood, or you can buy it online.

- **Plan your week.** Practice your new habits week by week. Sometimes when we think too far ahead, we get overwhelmed and respond by doing nothing, remaining with our old habits and then we stress with what to make for dinner because there's nothing in the fridge and you got home too late...and decide to order in because at this point you're starving. Generally, the easiest day to plan your week is on Sundays (although as of this writing, we are still living with COVID-19 and shelter in place, so it can be any day since most of us are home). There are a few parts to this:

  Go through your cupboard and refrigerator and keep a running list on your phone (or write it on paper) that you can check off while you are at the store. Do your food shopping and if your kids are old enough, enlist their help. As you run out of an item, make sure to put it on your list for the next shopping trip.

Think about what you want your week of meals to look like. Look at your calendar for the week. Do you have any dinner plans? How many times are you eating out? By planning ahead, you won't have to scramble at dinnertime to figure out what to make.

Prepare your vegetables. Chop and keep in separate containers. While it is true that once chopped, veggies start to lose their nutritional value, you also have to think about your stress levels when you don't plan and *do the best you can* (for those who are really crunched for time, there's always a place for frozen vegetables) without judgement.

Cook a few sweet potatoes (organic when possible), millet, brown rice, quinoa, pasta (of the variety I mentioned earlier) and keep in separate containers.

Have frozen wild salmon and free-range organic chicken or ground turkey in the freezer and take out to cook. You can also cook some chicken, grass fed burgers for a couple of days so that you can batch and know that lunch or dinner can be easily assembled. By being prepared it will be easier to put a meal together with your protein, healthy carbs, fiber and fat.

Live the 80/20 or 90/10 rule. Remember we don't want to be so restrictive (unless there is a health issue that requires you to be so) that we can't continue. When looking at your week, think about allowing yourself the indulgences that you once thought you had to cut out forever. Want chocolate? Have dark chocolate (80% or higher). Maybe it's a cocktail or cookies (homemade, of course). Re-frame your perspective so that you don't feel guilty. You'll find that eventually, your cravings for sugars, sweets and carbs will pretty much disappear as you provide your body with nutrient-dense food.

As a reminder, add in foods that your liver will thank you for, including asparagus, dandelions (or dandelion tea), garlic, nettle, and sea vegetables such as dulse, kelp, kombu (to name a few).

- **Intermittent fasting (IF).** The idea behind intermittent fasting is that you eat within a certain time window. Intuitively, that is how we eat, and the window can be anywhere from 8-12 hours and it's very individual with the caveat that you shouldn't eat past 7:00 or 8:00 p.m. Our body has a natural circadian rhythm of daytime, we eat; nighttime, we sleep. Rest and digest. It helps stabilize blood sugar, suppress inflammation and may improve blood pressure and cholesterol. If you have metabolic syndrome or type 2 diabetes, you may want to discuss this with your doctor and / or nutritionist.

- **Supplements.** In 2018, revenue from supplement sales in the US reached nearly $31 billion, reports Statista. It is projected to reach $61.8 billion by 2025. Globally, that number is expected to hit $210.3 billion by 2026, asserts GMD Research in an extensive September 2019 market report. That's a lot of money! The question is what do you need? Are you taking too much? Too little?

Is it working? Is your body absorbing the supplements? Until you understand what you need and perhaps have done a hair analysis or gut map, you may be wasting your money. Supplements are meant to supplement your nutrition, not to substitute. Can you benefit from probiotics? Absolutely! But what if you have SIBO? Your probiotics would be different than someone who doesn't have SIBO. How do you know if you even have SIBO? By connecting the dots through your symptoms and understanding your body, you can then work with your practitioner to determine what tests you need to get to the root causes of your symptoms. If you find that you are getting generic answers from your general practitioner, there are other options such as a functional nutritionist, functional doctor or naturopath—someone who will go deeper with you to determine what other types of tests you may need.

3. Self-Care

- **Exercise.** Your body needs to move. We weren't meant to sit in chairs all day. But what kind of movement? There are so many forms and you have to decide what you like. I always encourage my clients to try something new. You won't know unless you try. Also, how often and for how long? Do we really need to work out 1 hour a day? Not anymore. There are so many ways to have a more efficient workout including HIIT (high-intensity interval training) where, when done properly, can be effective in as little as 30 minutes. What about 10,000 steps a day? Is that real? Well, not really. Turns out that in 1964, a Japanese company made a device named Manpo-kei, which translates to "10,000 steps meter". The name was a marketing tool to get the population to walk more. According to I-Min Lee, a professor of epidemiology at the Harvard University T. H. Chan School of Public Health, the actual health benefits have never been validated by research. Yet, here we are, obsessed with Fitbits and watches reminding us to get our steps in. Now, don't get me wrong. There are many people who benefit from this type of structure. The point is not to feel as though you are missing out if you don't own one (FOMO) or if you haven't achieved the goal of 10,000 steps, because that will just increase your stress levels and we already know what stress does to our body.

> Listen to your body. There may be days that you need to take that 6-mile run or bike ride. Then there are days that you may feel that your body needs to rest. Maybe one week, it's all yoga. The key is to be consistent and honor that you are listening to your body. Decide how many days a week you want to work out. I have weeks where I may do Peloton twice, Barre class one day, one day lifting weights and the other days taking a walk. Then there are weeks where my body just wants to walk and do one day of weight training.

> Don't have time? Well, we know time is relative and we do have time. We all have the same 24 hours. *It's how we choose to spend our time.* Perspective.

Imagine this: you're single, out with friends at a party or a bar and you see a beautiful person and your heart starts to flutter. You flirt. That person asks you on a date. You want to say yes, but realize your schedule is packed for the next week. Chances are you that you will rearrange your calendar to go out with that person, right? If you can find time for that date, you can find time to exercise and you don't have to join a gym. You can look up workouts on YouTube or subscribe to an app.

- Let's do a little exercise around time. Humor me. We all have 168 hours in one week. Get a pen and fill in the chart below. How many hours you work, commute, sleep, exercise, kids, homework, run errands, laundry, cook, shop, date night...and all non-negotiables.

Activity	Hours
Work	
Commute	
Sleep	
Exercise	
Errands	

Kid related activities	
Household chores	
Any other non-negotiable	
Total	

Now, subtract that total from 168. What's your net number? See for yourself. You have more hours than you thought. So, where does the time go? If I were to guess, probably social media or TV, right? It's time to reframe how you look at your week and it's simple. Schedule it into your calendar. Put it in as an appointment to yourself. This is part of self-care and it's also a great productivity tool.

- **Journaling.** Let's face it. Our mental, emotional and spiritual health is important to our well-being. We are bombarded with so many messages and thoughts in our head that ruminate, and the energy stays stuck inside of us. By listening to our thoughts and using writing as a tool to connect to you, it becomes a great way to release the stagnant energy within. An article in *Positive Psychology* states that there are 83 benefits of journaling for depression, anxiety and stress. There are different ways to journal and again, as this is your journey, I encourage you to try them out.

  Bookend your day with gratitude and joy. This is the simplest and easiest way to change your perspective when things may not *seem* to be going your way. Take 15 minutes in the morning and write down 3 things you are grateful for. It could be as simple as being alive, having food to eat, to feeling gratitude for your financial health or for a person. In the evening, as you prepare for your bedtime routine, take out the same journal and write down 3 things that brought you joy that day. You may end up expanding this to 5 or 10 things. This awareness helps connect you and bring a smile to your face. No matter what is going on in the world, there is always something to be thankful for.

Another method is brain dumping. This works well if you wake up anxious and/or you can't shut your brain off before bed. Take out your journal and just do a brain dump where you write whatever you are thinking without structure (no paragraphs), without editing. This is stream of consciousness writing. By putting it down on paper, you are diffusing the energy that surrounded it in your brain.

- **Take an Epsom salt bath (or use magnesium flakes).** Magnesium helps the body to relax and reduce stress. Some researchers think that taking magnesium increases serotonin (the feel-good hormone) production. Most of us are low in this important mineral, so this is a relaxing way to add some into your body.

- **Find a creative outlet.** Think back to when you were a child. What did you love to do? Drawing? Puzzles? Dancing? Baking? Making jewelry? Listening to music or playing an instrument? Think about what brought you joy and if you have stopped engaging in those creative outlets, use this time to bring it back into your life. Just because we are adults does not mean we have to give up the simple joys of life (i.e. adult coloring books have become popular).

- **Practice better sleep habits.** This can include turning off your devices at least one hour before bed. Wear blue light glasses when you are on your electronic devices. Use a diffuser with calming essential oils to help you sleep. Make your bedroom your sanctuary.

When I first started working with people, a woman named Roberta came to one of the many "lunch and learns" that I held in people's kitchens. She was a Diet Mountain Dew fanatic. She had a lot of health issues, arthritis in her knees and needed to lose about forty pounds. When we got to this part of the exercise, she announced that she was going to give up her Diet Mountain Dew. Mouths dropped open, eyebrows raised, and no one believed her (she drank 2-3 a day).

"Wow? Can you really do that?"

"What are you going to drink instead?"

The skepticism and doubt were not uplifting, and I could tell by her body language (her shoulders dropped) that she was getting discouraged and already talking herself out of it.

"Ladies, let's shift this, give her some support and offer ideas that will be encouraging." There were nods of agreement and one suggestion was shared that this woman thought would work. "How about seltzer with lemon and lime squeezed in? Maybe instead of going cold turkey, you can exchange one Diet Mountain Dew a day with one seltzer and lemon/lime, and give yourself a week or two to wean yourself off of soda."

Bingo! The idea was brilliant. Roberta wouldn't have to worry if she "slipped" and had a soda; instead, she would incorporate adding in seltzer and slowly shift to replacing the soda with it entirely by the end of the second week. It ended up taking ten days for her to fully feel good not only about her decision, but also, that she even liked the taste of the seltzer and found that it got easier as the days passed.

Roberta went on to slowly shift her other habits of snacking, which were partly as a result of boredom. We asked her what she liked to do as a hobby that she could fill her time with when she was bored. She said she enjoyed making jewelry. Who knew? She decided to start making necklaces, which were beautiful, and she sold them. I still have one that I purchased from her. It's amazing what you can discover when you take the time to get connected, understand and take action. You may find a new business idea, hobby or passion to pursue once you are grounded.

WRITING EXERCISE
DIGEST AND DISCOVER

It's time to review all of your notes. After you read everything, close your eyes and ask yourself, *where do I want to start? What resonates with me right now?* This is really important. Listen closely. You may be surprised that it may have nothing to do with diet or losing weight and everything to do with stress and anxiety or something else. Write down what comes up for you. Then re-read what you wrote, close your eyes and ask yourself where you will start. Listen to that voice and you will hear a response that will be your answer. Remember, there is no right or wrong.

_____

_____

_____

_____

_____

_____

_____

_____

_____

_____

_____

_____

_____

_____

_____

_____

_____

_____

_____

At the end of each day, jot down your thoughts on what you added in and how it felt. Easy? Frustrating? Whatever that feeling was, ask yourself why you felt that way and what you think you could do to shift that.

_____

_____

_____

_____

_____

_____

_____

_____

_____

Another important component in this section is your
health history, any over-the-counter medications you
take regularly (or have taken in the past), and what other
modalities you have tried, because this will help enlighten
you as to when the story line of your health issues may
have developed. For instance, perhaps you had ear
infections as a child and were given antibiotics growing
up. Maybe you had surgery or a broken bone. Our bodies
are resilient, yet year after year, decade after decade,
there is only so much our bodies can handle (remember
the analogy about the army from an earlier chapter). Our
immune system doesn't weaken overnight. It had help and
now you have it in one place.

Fill out the information here. Not only will it help bring
awareness to you about your health; you'll have all the
information in one place so that when you do meet with a
doctor, nutritionist, or naturopath, you'll be able share the
information more easily.

Medical diagnosis

Diagnosis	
Current	
Past	
Date of Onset	

Diagnosis	
Current	
Past	
Date of Onset	

Diagnosis	
Current	
Past	
Date of Onset	

Diagnosis	
Current	
Past	
Date of Onset	

Past hospitalizations/surgeries

Hospitalization/ surgery	
Date	
Reason	

Hospitalization/ surgery	
Date	
Reason	

Hospitalization/ surgery	
Date	
Reason	

Hospitalization/ surgery	
Date	
Reason	

Antibiotics: Yes or no? How many times during your life?

Medications (and over the counter)

List all that you are taking.

Medication	
Dose	
Frequency	
Start Date	
Reason	

Medication	
Dose	
Frequency	
Start Date	
Reason	

Medication	
Dose	
Frequency	
Start Date	
Reason	

Medication	
Dose	
Frequency	
Start Date	
Reason	

Write down any new thoughts that may have come up while filling out these charts.

> **THE G.U.T. METHOD®**
> Get connected to your symptoms,
> what you're thinking, how you're feeling.

CHAPTER *12*

PROTECTING THE GIFTS IN YOUR GUT

....

"Success is not final, failure is not fatal:
it is the courage to continue that counts."

—*Winston S. Churchill*

....

Have you ever watched a baby learn how to walk? How do they know what to do? Why would they walk when their center of gravity is closer to the ground while they are crawling? What makes them get back up? Is it nature or nurture? Researchers have been studying this for 100 years, as documented in the piece fittingly titled "How Do You Learn to Walk? Thousands of Steps and Dozens of Falls Per Day". Infants accumulate massive amounts of practice; 12- to 19-month-olds averaged 2,368 steps and fell 17 times per hour!

Their brains aren't fully developed yet to tell them they can't do it. And parents encourage them constantly to keep trying. They record the moment. They clap and squeal with excitement and joy that their baby can walk. I remember those moments with each of my three kids. Had to get the camcorder out and ready for those first steps! And the younger they walk, the prouder the parent. They boast at how quickly their baby is learning.

Then that baby grows up. Their parents, teachers, peers, and society impose limitations. The baby is now an adult... you, reading this book. Somewhere along the way, the encouragement you once received turned into admonition about what you couldn't or shouldn't do. It was predicated on the assumption that you were wrong, and you needed to color inside the lines. This brings us back to our belief systems. They became ingrained in your subconscious and turned into your truth. They are all you know.

As a result, you may grow up second-guessing yourself or you may be so sure of what you think you know (some would call this being stubborn; I definitely fell into that category!), that you can't even fathom that there might be an alternative answer to a way of doing things. This may show up for you every January when you make a resolution to exercise more, or to go on a "diet" to lose those pesky ten pounds you gained during the holidays. It may look like you saying that this year, you will be nicer to your spouse. That you will listen more and work on your relationship.

It may look like you starting the year balancing your checkbook. Whatever it is, we all mean to take action, and we do...temporarily. But we fall back into our old habits.

I've mentioned those vampires sucking the energy out of you to feel better about themselves. We've all met and been surrounded by a few of those. The "woe is me," how everything is "happening to" them. They don't know why, and they complain and say, "But you don't understand." They unconsciously (or maybe consciously, depending on the person) manipulate you into feeling sorry for them and you spend the next hour trying to make them feel better, only to feel exhausted at the end and then have no energy to do what you want to or have to do.

We don't even realize that this is happening, and we keep going back for more.

It's exhausting. Now that you are connecting to yourself and understanding what you need, now is the time to truly trust yourself as you take action. Trust yourself to not have to ask anyone for validation on how you should be feeling or if you're doing *you* correctly. Because this journey is about you and what you need, and no one is going to know you better than yourself.

I have a memory of when I was young, before I was a teenager, when my mom would introduce me to people. I was quiet, and my mom would always say, "Oh, Sharon is just shy."

I believed that at the time. As I got older, I realized that it wasn't so much that I was shy; it was that I was an introvert. When my mother would announce that I'm shy, it told me that she knew me better than I knew myself.

I allowed it because I didn't know any better, because I didn't have the words to articulate what I was feeling.

As my life turned upside down during my divorce and when my son was diagnosed, I knew I had been given a chance to wake up and sever all those ties that bound me to what others thought of me. The one thing I had to do was shut out the world and learn to listen, tune in and trust myself. Much of that process consisted of letting go of my mom's voice—all those years of feeling 'less than' because of her very strong personality—and trusting that my inner voice knew what to do. I do want to acknowledge, and I've said this before, my mom did the best she could with what she knew…how to survive. I believe that all parents do the best they can with what they know, even if that is limited. We don't know what scars our parents have and what burdens they are carrying around with them and it's not fair to them or to us to make them wrong with our expectations. By surrendering and shifting your perception of how you think things should be to possibility of what could be, you create space to see what shows up. My mom and I have a new relationship. One that we've been working on for *years*. One that keeps evolving and expanding and I believe that this is happening because we are both engaging in the conversation. We are both working on listening better, not judging and releasing our perceived expectations. I have come to truly understand how her own life suffering shaped her thoughts and reality and who she became—who she thought she had to be in order to survive. I now love, appreciate and accept my mom. She is a human being who is also learning how to grow and be a better version of herself. That doesn't mean that those memories are gone. But I am not afraid to share what I think, to speak my truth. The fear and the triggers associated with them have dissipated. I am now aware of how I listen and can catch myself before I react.

My friend and colleague, Robin Meyers, a molecular geneticist and fear strategist, shares that fear is like a tattoo: While it is imprinted and difficult to remove, it is not impossible. They've been imprinted and with each layer that we peel away, the more resilient we become.

Taking action requires forgiveness of yourself and those whom you think have hurt you in some way but may not have had the tools to handle the situation at hand.

It requires self-compassion for yourself and constant reminders that it will never be perfect, but there will always be progress.

Taking action requires baby steps and room to dance along the way. Remember that illustration with the squiggly line to success? That's the dance. It's a reminder to enjoy the steps along the way so that you can stay present to who you are and how you want to show up in the world. It's about finding a point of balance that is unique to you. You want to find that sweet spot in the middle, that stillness, to find your truth and yourself.

What's missing really is *peace* and stillness within yourself. Resting within yourself so that you can find the *pieces* of your own soul that need nourishing. Sometimes we don't even realize the extent of that. That's why this section invites you to have so much compassion for yourself as you do others.

Most of my clients begin by going to the traditional western medicine route. When it doesn't work for them, then they start to move past it to understand that maybe it is bigger than that, and that is when they start to think that maybe it's time for them to look for a more holistic solution. To look at functional medicine and nutrition and see what other types of at home testing may be available that can get to the root of so many health concerns. And with that journey, as we work together, it will often go deeper and beyond the holistic journey to a more spiritual journey. You picked up this book for a reason. You have been guided here.

You are here because of all your choices to learn and grow. You may be at a crossroads in your path. No matter which direction you take, it will be the right one for you, *right now*, because all you have is the present. Trust yourself and know that each step will be revealed. You are ascending through your experiences. Your thoughts, beliefs, way of living are ready to expand, and your foundation will be rebuilt. As you ground yourself, you will have a greater knowing, a greater trust in yourself. You will have hope so that you can lift off to create whatever you're meant to create in this life. You don't have to know what that is right now. You've been given a blank canvas to design your next chapter, and while it may feel scary, you have an opportunity to paint your next masterpiece!

I've asked you to take a journey with me. One that may have created a crack in your belief systems, a shift in your story.

I remember the day that I had a huge *aha* moment. I wrote an article about it. Below is an excerpt:

e·piph·a·ny

As I was driving past a beautiful vista in my neighborhood, a song came on the radio. One I had heard many times before, but until now, had never really listened to the words.

It was overcast and it had just stopped raining and I could see a silver lining in the clouds as the sun tried desperately to save the day. Although I drive this route on a regular basis, something on this particular day made me pull over to stop and admire the beauty that surrounded me.

My mind went from thought to thought as I reflected on my recent divorce and how my three teenagers and I had grown over the last four years as a result. We were lucky, a term you don't ordinarily associate with divorce. And I was happy. Until I had reached that point, I don't even think I realized what that meant in its real sense. Externally, sure, I was happy the day I graduated college, procured my first job, had a baby, etc., but those fleeting moments would dissipate after the initial euphoria wore off, until I was left with the emptiness again, searching for the next moment that would lift my spirits.

As I sat there contemplating these thoughts, I realized the radio was on, and a song that I heard but had never really listened to before had started to play. Natasha Bedingfield's "Unwritten" filled the quiet air in my car. What was once static background music transformed into a strong wave of energy and sent sensations that filled me to the core.

Her lyrics talked about reaching for something that was so close that you could almost taste it, but it was still in the distance. She sang about releasing your inhibitions and feeling things like the rain on your skin. And that only you could be the one to feel it. No one could feel it for you, only you can experience it. She was singing and asking me to open my arms wide and allow life in, allow myself to live on my terms.

"No one else can speak the words on your lips. Drench yourself in words unspoken, live your life with arms wide open. Today is where your book begins..."

Why today? Why now was I paying attention to this particular song that I had heard so many times before? Why was I having a physical reaction to this song? Was it that I was now ready to receive new information? Was what I was feeling something new, or had it just lay there dormant, waiting to be awoken? Was the static in my head clearing also? The silver lining? Were these all signs that I was finally seeing the proverbial elephant in the room?

As the chorus started to repeat, the words reverberated, and I started crying. I was so overwhelmed with emotion.

Years of it that had built up and was finally being released. All this from a song. And that was when I had the epiphany (one of many to come). These words, this song, was a metaphor for my present life. It was what I needed to hear at that moment, at that time. I had released so much these past few years, and this was my turning point. No one else can feel it for you or do it for you or speak for you. I had been so shut down and was surviving, each moment, each day, each year. Live your life with arms wide open... my divorce, my book, was just beginning. The universe was sending me a sign. In fact, it had been sending me signs for years, but I was ignoring them. Not anymore.

Things happen for a reason to all of us, yet only a few really understand this. We go through each day, not paying attention to the seemingly mundane things—a song, a silver lining in the sky, a beautiful, majestic field in the distance—and we miss those signs that can have the biggest impact on our lives. I wondered how many I had missed in the past. But then again, the past is the past, and I was here in the present, now suddenly aware of so much more and looking forward to what today brought and what the future had in store.

I chose at that moment to lock that door to the past and to appreciate what I had now. And as I looked back out at the field, the sun had driven the clouds away and was now shining; its rays beaming everywhere, as was the smile on my face that stayed with me as I put the car in drive and moved forward with my life.

As I sit here writing these words, my hope for you is that you, too, will live your life with arms wide open and write the words for your own book, because you deserve to live a life of joy, hope, empowerment and courage, while learning to be vulnerable and honest and true to yourself, your soul, and to your loved ones and those you surround yourself with.

This article about my epiphany opened a new door for me. It offered me possibilities of looking at situations with a different lens. It made me realize that I had a choice and that I needed to do some work. I needed to be really honest, raw and vulnerable. Sometimes it's just easier to live in the discomfort because we're comfortable there and taking a deep look into our souls is painful. The shame and guilt that surrounds us is bountiful. And the failure that we feel, well, you can't really put a price on that, can you? However, if you look at pain, so many times beauty can be born from it. After all, how does a lotus grow if not for the mud from which it was born?

One Life in This Body

I've asked you to take a journey. To rediscover who you are, what you feel. To get connected to you and become aware of your symptoms, your thoughts, to understand what that means in the scope of your life and to take action. To tune in and trust yourself.

I've asked you not to participate in groups where you feel you are comparing yourself or needing validation because the truth is that you have those answers within.

With awareness, so that you don't sucked into the vampire's lair (do vampires even have a lair? I don't know, but it sounds good!), because it's so easy to get hooked and obsessed. Before you know it, hours disappear, you didn't get what you want done, then you kick yourself because you told yourself that you were only going to stay on social media for thirty minutes today, not an hour. Which adds to anxiety, more self-loathing, which leads to gut issues.

We need to slow down. We have one life in this body, and we need to hit the pause button and re-evaluate what it is we truly want. That starts with you and your number one asset: your health. Without it, what do you really have?

Don't let your fears hold you back. Fear, after all really means False Evidence Appearing Real.

Start putting your support system together. Fill it with people who will cheer you on and encourage you to continue. When you find the right person/people to help hold you accountable, miracles happen. Their positive energy and belief in your success will give you the space to be you. They will encourage you and remind you why you are doing this. They will pick you up when you get stuck or frustrated and won't let you quit when you're feeling down. They will allow you to feel what you are feeling and remind you of what is working, of where you are from when you started and, most importantly, why you are doing this. What I've noticed most with my clients and myself is that the hardest part is the self-talk. It's our minds, the psychology of the years of shit we've been feeding it both consciously and unconsciously. It's the part of our mind that urges, "Warning, warning, do not go there! You'll be sorry. You know what happens every time you try, so don't."

It's the part of our mind that asks you who you think you are to think that this time you'll be successful. Who you think you are to imagine that there's a life filled with joy, a life where you don't have to have a closet filled with fat jeans or have to run to the bathroom because you have IBS or where every other commercial on TV is a drug that rattles off a list of side effects and possible stroke or death.

Yet, you know. You know, deep down that you want to take that leap, past the fear of failing, of being disappointed, of what people may think of you, of what you'll think of yourself. Do you deserve it? Of course, you do!

Your thoughts didn't just occur overnight. But now, thanks to awareness, you can take it one day at a time, knowing that the more you practice, the easier it will get.

The more I focused on adding in healthy foods, the less obsessed I felt. I promised myself I would not get on a scale and would instead, just think about how I felt when I put on my pants. Note: I had jeans in four different sizes. I promised myself that I would do it slowly. Add in a healthy vegetable and swap out the sleeve of fat-free cookies for an apple with organic peanut butter or celery or even dark chocolate. Drink more water.

I also reminded myself that I don't live in the woods. I don't eat bamboo shoots and leaves, and I don't have to subscribe to one "diet". I love going out to dinner and you know, there are times that I am just dying for a burger (grass-fed whenever possible). My body would be craving red meat and I would let myself enjoy it because I listened to my body and what it was asking for. I'd sit and chew and savor it. And that would be it.

Part of having that freedom is not only having gone through the G.U.T. Method, but also, getting the right tests to get to the root of lingering symptoms.

When you drive a car and use your GPS to get from point A to point B, if you make a wrong turn, the voice that you hear from the GPS system doesn't yell at you, does it? Does it say, "You dummy, why can't you follow instructions? Why did you make a left when I told you to make a right?"

No, instead, it says, "Recalculating," and it redirects you to get you back on track. You didn't have to call or text your spouse, sibling, or friend and ask them what to do. You didn't have to go on Facebook and ask someone in the group what to do. How would they know anyway? They may never have taken that route before and may live in a different country.

You have your own navigation system. It's intuitive... Y.O.U.

My goal with this book is to help you begin your healing process. My objective is to share this knowledge because if you are anything like me, you want answers and hope and a knowing that you are not crazy. For some, this book may be enough. For others who need testing or help with accountability, I encourage you to seek assistance. Either way, this book and your participation with the journaling has created YOUR manual for your body so that you have a reference to go back to when you feel stuck or need to revisit or revise a section. After all, we are all dynamic human beings and if we allow ourselves, we will bend and flow like a willow tree.

Regardless of which path you choose, knowing that there is something bigger out there for you to consider, is hope enough to know that you, or someone you love does not have to become a statistic. That you can truly design your lifestyle, by following your inner guidance system. When there is no resistance, your body and your mind are in alignment, then you know it's right for you. That's the goal, knowing what is right for you. Remember, you are the one living in your body. No one knows you better than you know yourself.

When I had my epiphany that day, many years ago, I never imagined I'd be where I am now. I never imagined how life could be full of such possibilities or that I would truly love what I did. I never imagined that when I used to play school with friends when I was a kid and I was the teacher that I would grow up and being in a profession where I get to be of service and educate. I never imagined that this book would ever be published, let alone written.

I remember when my twins were born. At the time, there weren't many parenting books on how to raise twins or what to do during those first few months, especially when you had a 4-year-old toddler running around. I remember lamenting to a good friend who worked for a large publishing house about how I wished there was a book like *What to Expect When You're Expecting* on how to raise twins. I was overwhelmed, hormones raging, happy one minute, depressed the next, laughing one minute, crying the next. Overwhelmed with their feed and sleeping schedules and how to keep my 4-year-old happy. And I said to her, "I have to write a book. I can do this," and she encouraged me.

I got excited. I wrote the introduction. The first chapter, the whole outline. At this point, my twins were almost 2 years old, and I had gotten parenting down and felt great. My friend read the chapters and the outline and loved it. She introduced me to an agent who loved it. I remember thinking, *wow, it's happening. I'm going to write a book and be on national TV and help other moms with twins and triplets get through it (this was way before Facebook)*!

Then the agent called. A doctor was writing a book on raising twins and, well, she had the credentials. Really? Did she even have twins? No. She was a pediatrician. Then he asked me to put a market analysis together for my book and why it should be published. I froze. My elation quickly squashed like a bug. Marketing analysis? What the heck was that? Where do I start? He told me to research it and get back to him without offering any help.

I hung up the phone, crushed. I remember feeling paralyzed and not knowing what to do next. I couldn't ask for help because I was raised not to. I was raised to stay quiet and not color outside the lines. When my friend asked how it was going, I didn't tell here the whole truth or ask her for help. I was embarrassed. I felt like I had failed. I said they were going to publish a pediatrician's book instead of mine. I could have asked her for help, but that would have made me weak and an imposter and who was I to think I could do this anyway. I had a banking and finance degree. What did I know about writing and publishing a book?

And the dream died.

If I could go back to my 32-year-old self now, I would kick her in the ass and tell her to get off her high horse and do it. To believe in herself, that her credentials as a mom of twins were enough and to not be embarrassed and to ask for help. But I believe that things happen for a reason. And at the time, a seed was planted. A seed of wanting to help. To be of service. To educate. It was unconscious at the time because I was still unconsciously incompetent (I'm beginning to like that phrase!).

I still had a lot to learn. I still had an ego that needed taming. Anger that needed to be diffused in a healthy way. Sadness that needed to be resolved. Mommy issues, which I've shared a little of and...well, that's a whole other book (with a happy ending).

Truth be told, who knows where we'd be, how my son would be doing now, or any of us, if I had taken a different path. I wasn't meant to write that book at that time. I was on a journey, and so are you.

Now, this is your time. It's not a coincidence that Brené Brown, Mel Robbins, and Rachel Hollis are at the forefront of a major movement that tells us we have the answers within. Oprah has been talking about this for years. You can dare greatly, and stop apologizing and counting down, and own who you are.

My son was my wake-up call. While at the time, I couldn't see the trees through the forest because I was in it just trying to make it through another day, I eventually surrendered my fears, my anguish, and my anger to the universe.

We are all on a journey. I heard a phrase once that really stuck with me: "We are all spiritual beings having a human experience." At the time, I wondered what the heck that meant. It would take me years to understand energy and how our thoughts create our reality and how epigenetics confirms that we do have the power to change our DNA.

We are living a life now that you couldn't imagine being remotely possible just a decade ago. With that, we are growing and expanding. At the end of the long day, we all have choices. Free will. Like Morpheus said in "The Matrix," no one can tell you what the matrix is, you have to see it and feel it for yourself.

Something inside of you is calling out to you to wake up. To take your power back and to realize that you have infinite possibilities. All you have to do is say yes. Say yes and take one step at a time. Know that while that mountain seems huge and you can't see it, you don't have to. You just need to see the first step and the rest will reveal itself.

You must take back control of your health. Your power starts from within. You need that oxygen mask so that you can make it up that mountain and bring others with you.

Keep choosing. Keep going. Keep thriving.

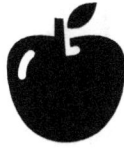

WHAT'S NEXT?

With your newfound knowledge of The G.U.T. Method and design of a blueprint for your health, your life, for more resources, visit www.thegutmethod.com.

Stay connected. Continue to understand, tune in, and trust yourself to take action. Transform your life.

REFERENCES

Ackerman, Courtney. "83 Benefits of Journaling for Depression, Anxiety, and Stress."

Positivepsychology.com. April 28, 2020.

https://positivepsychology.com/benefits-of-journaling/

Adolph, Karen E., Whitney G. Cole, Meghana Komati, Jessie S. Garciaguirre, Daryaneh

American College of Gastroenterology.
Irritable Bowel Syndrome.

https://gi.org/topics/irritable-bowel-syndrome/#:~:text=In%20the%20United%20States%2C%20it%20is%20estimated%20that%2010%20to15,seen%20by%20primary%20care%20physicians

American Diabetes Association. Economic Costs of Diabetes in the U.S. in 2017. Diabetes Care. 2018 May;41(5):917-928. doi: 10.2337/dci18-0007. Epub 2018 Mar 22.

Anxiety and Depression Association of America. https://adaa.org/about-adaa/press-room/facts-statistics

Asprey, Dave. *The Bulletproof Diet Book*. New York, New York: Rodale Books, 2014.

Badaly, Jesse M. Lingeman, Gladys Chan, and Rachel B. Sotsky. How Do You Learn to Walk? Thousands of Steps and Dozens of Falls Per Day. Psychol Sci. Author manuscript; available in PMC 2013 Oct 19. Psychol Sci. 2012; 23(11): 1387–1394.

Banting, William. Letter on Corpulence, Addressed to the Public (Third Edition). *Wiley Online Library.* First published: March 1993.

https://doi.org/10.1002/j.1550-8528.1993.tb00605.x

Barbour KE, Helmick CG, Boring M, Brady TJ. Vital Signs: Prevalence of Doctor-Diagnosed Arthritis and Arthritis-Attributable Activity Limitation—United States, 2013–2015. *Morb Mortal Wkly Rep* 2017;66:246–253.

doi: http://dx.doi.org/10.15585/mmwr.mm6609e1External.

Burch, Noel. Four Learning Stages Model. Gordon Training International. 2016.

Dweck, Carol. *Mindset.* New York, New York: Ballantine Books, 2007.

Egeberg A, Hansen PR, Gislason GH, and Thyssen JP. Clustering of autoimmune diseases in patients with rosacea. *J Am Acad Dermatol.* 2016 Apr;74(4):667-72.e1. doi: 10.1016/j.jaad.2015.11.004. Epub 2016 Jan 30.

General Psychiatry. Research: Effects of regulating intestinal microbiota on anxiety symptoms: A systematic review doi 10. 1136/gpsych-2019-100056.

Gershoff, Stanley N. Jean Mayer 1920–1993. *The Journal of Nutrition*, Volume 131, Issue 6, June 2001, Pages 1651–1654, https://doi.org/10.1093/jn/131.6.1651

GMD Research. "North America Nutritional Supplements Market by Ingredient, Product Form, Application, End-user, Supplement Classification, Distribution Channel, and Country 2019-2026: Trend Forecast and Growth Opportunity." September 2019.

https://www.researchandmarkets.com/reports/4845595/north-america-nutritional-supplements-market-by?utm_source=BW&utm_medium=PressRelease&utm_code=73k2q5&utm_campaign=1303606+-+North+America%27s+%2461.8+Billion+Nutritional+Supplements+Market%2c+2019+to+2025&utm_exec=joca220prd

Gundry, Steven R. Dr. *The Plant Paradox*. New York, New York: Harper Wave, April 25, 2017.

Hootman JM, Helmick CG, Barbour KE, Theis KA, Boring MA. Updated projected prevalence of self-reported doctor-diagnosed arthritis and arthritis-attributable activity limitation among US adults, 2015-2040. *Arthritis Rheumatol*. 2016;68(7):1582–1587. doi: 10.1002/art.39692. PubMed PMID: 27015600.

Kessler, David A. *The End of Overeating*. New York, New York: Rodale Press, 2010.

Lee, So-Yeon, Eun Lee, Yoon Mee Park, and Soo-Jong Hong. Microbiome in the Gut-Skin Axis in Atopic Dermatitis. *Allergy Asthma Immunol Res*. 2018 Jul; 10(4): 354–362.

Published online 2018 Feb 26. doi: 10.4168/aair.2018.10.4.354

Lipton, Bruce. "The Wisdom of Your Cells." Sounds True CDs. 2016.

MacDonald, Ann. Using the Relaxation Response to Reduce Stress. Harvard Healthy Publishing. November 10, 2010.

https://www.health.harvard.edu/blog/using-the-relaxation-response-to-reduce-stress-20101110780

Miguel-Kergoat, Sophie, Veronique Azais-Braesco, Britt Burton-Freeman, and Marion M. Hetherington "Effects of chewing on appetite, food intake and gut hormones: A systematic review and meta-analysis." *Physiology and Behavior.* Volume 151, November 2015, Pages 88-96.

https://doi.org/10.1016/j.physbeh.2015.07.017

Miller, Lee J. and Wei Lu. These Are the World's Healthiest Nations. Bloomberg.com. February 24, 2019.

https://www.bloomberg.com/news/articles/2019-02-24/spain-tops-italy-as-world-s-healthiest-nation-while-u-s-slips

Moloney RD, Johnson AC, O'Mahony SM, Dinan TG, Greenwood-Van Meerveld

B, Cryan JF. Stress and the Microbiota-Gut-Brain Axis in Visceral Pain: Relevance to Irritable Bowel Syndrome. *CNS Neurosci Ther.* 2016 Feb;22(2):102-17. doi: 10.1111/cns.12490. Epub 2015 Dec 10.

Mull, Amanda. "What 10,000 Steps Will Really Get You." The Atlantic. May 31, 2019.

https://www.theatlantic.com/health/archive/2019/05/10000-steps-rule/590785/

National Institute of Allergy and Infectious Diseases. Autoimmune Diseases.

https://www.niaid.nih.gov/diseases-conditions/autoimmune-diseases

Nelson, Portia. *There's a Hole in My Sidewalk*. New York, New York: Atria Books/Beyond Words, 1994.

Oppenheimer, Gerald M. and J. Daniel Benrubi. McGovern's Senate Select Committee on Nutrition and Human Needs Versus the: Meat Industry on the Diet-Heart Question (1976–1977). *Am J Public Health*. 2014 January; 104(1): 59–69. Published online 2014 January. doi: 10.2105/AJPH.2013.301464

Sargen, Molly, and Daniel Utter. "Biological Roles of Water: Why is water necessary for life?" Science in the News/managed by Harvard University. September 26, 2019.

http://sitn.hms.harvard.edu/uncategorized/2019/biological-roles-of-water-why-is-water-necessary-for-life/

Sharma VK, M R, S V, Subramanian SK, Bhavanani AB, Madanmohan, Sahai A, Thangavel D. Effect of Fast and Slow Pranayama Practice on Cognitive Functions in

Healthy Volunteers. J Clin Diagn Res. 2014 Jan;8(1):10-3. doi: 10.7860/JCDR/2014/7256.3668. Epub 2013 Nov 18.

Stempel, Anthony. "Bayer's Monsanto pleads guilty to illegal Hawaii pesticide spraying." *Reuters.* November 22, 2019.

https://www.reuters.com/article/us-bayer-monsanto-plea-hawaii/bayers-monsanto-pleads-guilty-to-illegal-hawaii-pesticide-spraying-idUSKBN1XW21N

Thailand Medical News. Rosacea and Small Intestinal Bacterial Overgrowth (SIBO). October 9, 2018.

https://www.thailandmedical.news/pages/health/rosacea-and-small-intestinal-bacterial-overgrowth-sibo

Weis, Emma, and Rajani Katta. Diet and Rosacea. *Dermatology Practical and Conceptual.* 2017 Oct; 7(4): 31–37. Published online 2017 Oct 31. doi: 10.5826/dpc.0704a08

World Health Organization. https://www.who.int

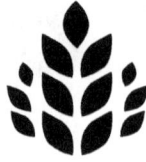

ACKNOWLEDGEMENTS

I never imagined two years ago when I first started writing this book, that the day would come for actually printing it. Getting all my thoughts on to paper was a feat in and of itself, and I am thankful to my writing mentor, Maggie McReynolds, for helping me focus on my story and my readers. You stuck with me when I was cranky, feeling discouraged that this would never end, and frustrated when there were gaps and I stared at a blank page wanting to give up!

Thank you to my editor and PR partner, Candi S. Cross of You Talk I Write, for organizing my chapters, reminding me of my timeframe, and taking me to the finish line. I knew when we met that you would be involved in this process...*you had me at hello!*

There are so many people I've met over the last few years who have unknowingly helped me on my journey. Thank you to all of my mentors and coaches over the years. Some were central and in the forefront and others didn't even realize how they impacted my education and goals, from my mentors at FDN: Reed Davis, Brandon Molle, Brendan Vermiere, Whitney Morgan, to the other

FDN'ers who are on this journey—this was a huge missing component to my work and I thank you for all that you do. To Kendra Perry and Anna Lubaszka, thank you for your mentorship and support with my hair analysis training!

Thank you to Tricia Brouk, mentor and friend. You helped me find my voice and I know our work is not yet done!

Thank you, Michael Roderick, for helping to create my framework and the acronym for G.U.T. Your insights helped me see things from a whole new perspective...one that continues to evolve.

Thank you to all of my clients who I've had the privilege to serve and help heal, and to my readers who continue to inspire me as we all take back control of our health.

A big thank you to all of my friends old and new... from childhood (yes, Iris, that's you) to adulthood: Sharon, Karen, Sheryl, Lori, Susan, Leslie, Nancy, Katie, Linda, Kate, and the countless others, you know who you are and I know there are so many! Your friendship and support have been a great source of comfort and strength.

Thank you to Robin Myers. Who knew when we met at Speaker Salon that our friendship would lead us to create our "Lunch and Life" show together and so much more. I'm excited for what the future holds.

Thank you, Mike Schonberg, for entering my life and for being on this journey as we learn, grow and expand together.

Thank you to my family. Mom, your story, your experiences, helped shaped who I was and who I am. Your own personal growth has helped me truly understand that we are all human beings with the capacity to forgive, grow, love and accept one another as we are. You and Dad created a legacy for the whole family through your love, tenacity and perseverance and I feel blessed for our entire family and for you.

Dad, you left us too soon. There are so many things I would say to you now that I didn't have time to share, but I know you are watching out over all of us, with that tremendous smile from ear to ear, wanting us all to be happy. Thank you for coming to America to create a better life for all of us.

Adina, what can I say? *I am so blessed.* You are not just my sister, you are my best friend, my soulmate, my rock. You have always been there in good times and bad and you will always be my partner in crime! The love I feel for you, Jeff, Justin and Tyler, keeps expanding. Thank you.

To my former husband, Bill, I am grateful. Life can throw many lemons and yet, we have managed to make lemonade by putting our kids first and raising them with love.

Lastly, this book and my life wouldn't be what it is today without my children: Evan, Zach and Nicki. Zach, your diagnosis was truly a blessing in disguise. It opened up the door to a new way of thinking, a new way of being and showing up in the world that has brought so much joy and light into our hearts. This has been the greatest gift. My heart overflows with love for the three of you, and not only the relationship we have, but also, the relationship that you have with each other. I continue to learn from you and look forward to seeing how each of our stories and journeys continue to unfold. Thank you for letting me be your mom. I love you.

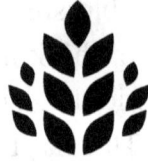

ABOUT THE AUTHOR

Sharon Holand Gelfand, a functional diagnostic nutritionist, coach and speaker, transforms the lives of health-minded professional women, who are stressed out and overwhelmed, by getting to the root of their most common health complaints with specific testing, not guessing. She incorporates the results with their symptoms to find the missing pieces of their health puzzle so they can reclaim their health and their lives.

When her son was diagnosed with Crohn's disease, instead of accepting the status quo, Sharon tackled his condition head-on. This led her to a breakthrough career change and sent her to graduate school, where she completed an M.S. in Applied Clinical Nutrition. Sharon works with individuals virtually, and takes her expertise to stages, panels, and workshops to share her very important message of healing with the world. Clients include Sysco, Priceline.com, New York Athletic Club, Global Community Charter School, and HGAR, among others.

Sharon is also the creator of The G.U.T. Method®, a three-step system to empower others to take back control of their health by getting connected to symptoms, understanding what that means to one's life so the right actions can be taken for ultimate healing.

The G.U.T. Method®: Secrets Beyond Your Plate for Healthier, More Energetic Living is Sharon's debut book.